STATISTICAL BASES OF REFERENCE VALUES IN LABORATORY MEDICINE

STATISTICS: Textbooks and Monographs

A Series Edited by

D. B. Owen, Founding Editor, 1972–1991

W. R. Schucany, Coordinating Editor
Department of Statistics
Southern Methodist University
Dallas, Texas

R. G. Cornell, Associate Editor
for Biostatistics
University of Michigan

W. J. Kennedy, Associate Editor
for Statistical Computing
Iowa State University

A. M. Kshirsagar, Associate Editor
for Multivariate Analysis and
Experimental Design
University of Michigan

E. G. Schilling, Associate Editor
for Statistical Quality Control
Rochester Institute of Technology

Additional Volumes in Preparation

STATISTICAL BASES OF REFERENCE VALUES IN LABORATORY MEDICINE

EUGENE K. HARRIS
JAMES C. BOYD

University of Virginia
Charlottesville, Virginia

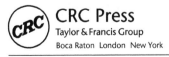

CRC Press
Taylor & Francis Group
Boca Raton London New York

CRC Press is an imprint of the
Taylor & Francis Group, an **informa** business

CRC Press
Taylor & Francis Group
6000 Broken Sound Parkway NW, Suite 300
Boca Raton, FL 33487-2742

First issued in paperback 2019

© 1995 by Taylor & Francis Group, LLC
CRC Press is an imprint of Taylor & Francis Group, an Informa business

ISBN-13: 978-0-8247-9339-5 (hbk)
ISBN-13: 978-0-367-40167-2 (pbk)

Visit the Taylor & Francis Web site at
http://www.taylorandfrancis.com

and the CRC Press Web site at
http://www.crcpress.com

In memory of
George Z. Williams, M.D. (1907–1994),
a leader in laboratory medicine
and a good friend

PREFACE

The interpretation of any measurement of an individual depends on the existence of a body of relevant information to which that measurement may be referred for comparison. This axiom is perhaps most evident in the clinical use of laboratory tests where "reference" values or their predecessors, "normal" values, have been called upon by generations of physicians to help them interpret the results of biochemical or physiological tests of patients. Indeed, the creation and use of reference information in medical practice, particularly in the diagnosis of disease, must go back to the very beginnings of medicine. Nevertheless, only within the last half-century has there developed what might be called a science of reference values: a body of knowledge, both theoretical and empirical, concerning the collection, description, analysis, and application of such information.

Since reference values reflect biological sources of variation (as well as measurement errors), this body of knowledge includes concepts and methods of biostatistics. In this book, we

v

identify topics that we believe are important aspects of reference values in laboratory medicine. Within each subject area, we discuss the current and potential uses of biostatistics. Chapters 1 to 9 group themselves into three general but overlapping categories. Chapters 1 to 5 review methods for deriving population-based reference ranges or other indices involving all three components of variation combined: biological variation among and within persons and analytical variation due to measurement error. Chapters 6 and 7 direct attention to within-subject variation, including both biological and analytical components. Chapters 8 and 9 focus on the analytical component while necessarily relating this to within-subject biological variation.

Clinical chemists, pathologists, and clinicians constitute our primary target audience, although biostatisticians interested in or already working on problems related to laboratory medicine will find this a useful reference. Some elementary statistical material has been included in the earlier chapters to help introduce the chemist or clinician to the subsequent methodology. Other sections contain statistical material probably too advanced for most readers in our primary audience. We hope, however, that at least they will "catch the music if not the lyrics" of these sections, and that the interest of biostatisticians will be maintained.

During the decade of the 1980s, and even earlier, national and international associations of clinical chemists published recommended guidelines for the successive steps in the process of obtaining 95 percent reference ranges. They were particularly concerned with the issues of selection of reference subjects, rules for subjects' treatment prior to and during collection of blood specimens, and the handling of the specimens before analysis. We mention these guidelines briefly in Chapter 1, citing in particular the sequence of reports by the Expert Panel of the International Federation for Clinical Chemistry. We also step through the debate in the 1960s about whether or not hospital patients should be used to provide "normal" ranges. In principle, this point of contention is no longer a real problem .

within the context of reference ranges since patients can form reference populations of their own. However, the argument raised questions about the real purpose of reference ranges and the effects of heterogeneity among reference subjects. The latter, at least, is a subject to which statistical ideas and methods can make an important contribution.

Arguments over whether to use parametric or nonparametric methods to derive reference limits have occupied space in the clinical chemistry literature for well over 20 years. In Chapter 2, we try to deal fully and fairly with the various methods proposed. In the end, we suggest either of two procedures: the nonparametric Harrell-Davis bootstrap method or a Box-Cox transform followed, if necessary, by a second transform to eliminate residual kurtosis.

Two areas not well covered in the guidelines of the International Federation for Clinical Chemistry are the number of subjects to include in a determination of reference ranges and criteria for deciding when to produce separate ranges for different subgroups of a population. These topics have been more thoroughly studied in recent research, as described in Chapter 3. Also included in this chapter are methods for deciding whether or not to reject outliers in a sample of reference values.

Sample size is important not only to manufacturers required to determine reference ranges associated with the analytical materials they produce and distribute, but also to user laboratories which must validate the manufacturers' published ranges in their own clinical practice. The problem of assuring valid transference of reference ranges from manufacturer to user laboratories within the United States deserves more serious attention than it has yet received. Chapter 3 ends with a brief consideration of some simple statistical guidelines that may be useful in dealing with this problem.

Multivariate reference regions are still considered statistical curiosities by most clinical chemists. One reason for this may be that in healthy persons the concentrations of different biochemical analytes are generally independent of each other. Even in this case, however, the multivariate reference region would be more desirable than multiple univariate reference ranges because of its greater specificity against false positives. In disease, otherwise independent variables are often highly correlated, and the diagnostic process may then benefit from multivariate regions derived from former patients with these diseases. However, the most useful set of biochemical tests to include in a multivariate index depends on the specific diseases to be distinguished, as shown by experience with discriminant functions in differential diagnosis. The statistical background minimally necessary for understanding multivariate reference regions and indices is presented in Chapter 4 together with a discussion and application of some relatively simple tests for dealing with multivariate outliers.

The concentrations of biochemical substances in blood are functions of physiological activities that change with age. This dependence on age has usually been recognized only in terms of broad age groups, such as pediatric reference ranges or reference ranges in the elderly. In women, pre- and postmenopausal ranges for cholesterol and alkaline phosphatase have been suggested. Only recently, however, has the clinical chemistry literature begun to recognize that many, perhaps most, biochemical analytes change continuously over the life span of healthy individuals, although at a faster rate during certain age intervals than others. During the past decade, various statistical methods, parametric and nonparametric, for determining age-specific reference ranges have been reported in the biostatistics literature. These are described in Chapter 5. Also included is a discussion of problems associated with the use of longitudinal biochemical data to estimate conditional reference ranges in rapidly changing processes during pregnancy or early childhood.

Chapter 6 focuses on the ratio of within-person to between-persons variances as a means of judging the utility of the population-based reference limits in long-term monitoring of apparently healthy individuals. The central role of within-person variance in this activity is further demonstrated through mathematical models discussed in Chapter 7. This chapter goes on to review some time series models appropriate for patient management after treatment, combining estimation of population parameters with Bayesian forecasting of serial laboratory results in individual patients.

Reference values, like all biochemical assays carried out in a clinical laboratory, are rarely completely accurate. That is, except by chance, the reported value will not agree exactly with the concentration of analyte contained in the specimen subjected to analysis. Over many years, improved analytical methods and vigorous quality control programs have greatly reduced analytical imprecision and bias within and among clinical laboratories. Nevertheless, the question of appropriate analytical goals for clinical laboratories continues to be discussed and argued within the profession. The effect of inaccuracy on the reliability of reference limits and other medical decision points clearly relates to our central concern with the statistical bases of reference values. In Chapter 8, we review the uses of biostatistical models and methods to help resolve problems in setting standards for the analysis of normally occurring blood constituents. Chapter 9 extends this review to the area of analytical standards for the assay of exogenous substances in blood, specifically therapeutic drugs. Here the therapeutic range, particularly the upper limit of that range, becomes the reference value for clinicians and clinical laboratories.

In the last chapter, Chapter 10, we project the likely effects of some current directions in laboratory medicine, and medicine as a whole, on the definition and use of reference values. We consider in particular the rapid progress being made in four areas: computer-based integration of patient records, laboratory automation (especially robotics), medical telecommunications, and molecular genetics. In our view, these forces will have at least two important effects on reference values. They will stimulate the use of patient-specific predictive values to guide in interpreting serial results (Chapter 7). In addition, they will encourage the development of outcome-based reference cutpoints that may differ considerably from conventional 95 percent reference limits. Such cutpoints have already been determined for serum cholesterol as a risk factor in coronary heart disease. These are discussed in some detail in Chapters 1 and 8.

Many sets of real data and examples of calculations have been included. We hope that this will make the book useful not only as a source of information on the statistical bases of reference values in laboratory medicine, but also in training students and residents in clinical biochemistry and pathology.

Finally, we would like to express our deep thanks to those who have encouraged us in this work. The first author especially remembers with gratitude the welcome extended to him almost 30 years ago by pathologists George Williams and Ernest Cotlove to participate as a statistician in their pioneering research on components of variance in serial studies of biochemical constituents in healthy individuals. Roger Gilbert, for many years an innovative leader in the College of American Pathologists, was very kind to invite him to take part in the 1976 Aspen conference on analytical goals in clinical chemistry, thereby enabling him to meet others concerned with this problem in this country and abroad. To Callum Fraser and Per Hyltoft Petersen for vigorous discussions of many topics in clinical biochemistry over the years, and to Michael Healy for never-failing statistical mentorship and encouragement, E.K.H. remains deeply grateful.

We have received invaluable support from the Department of Pathology at the University of Virginia Health Sciences Center, including outstanding secretarial assistance from Debra Reed. We are also indebted to Mary Johnston Schubert, Dr. Robin A. Felder, and Dr. Doris M. Haverstick in the Department of Pathology, and Dr. Marguerite C. Lippert in the Department of Urology for providing the data on prostate-specific antigen used in one of the examples.

Eugene K. Harris
James C. Boyd

CONTENTS

1

SOME HISTORY OF REFERENCE VALUES

1

1.1 INTRODUCTION

In this chapter, we sketch rather lightly some of the different points of view, the investigative methods, and the emerging ideas of the past 40 years' search for reference values needed in medical practice. Although clinical needs have always been the prime movers in this search, statistical methods were involved from the beginning, as in all studies of human variation. Both medical and statistical practice have changed considerably during these years, influenced by advances in research and technology. But reference values, whatever form they may assume in one clinical situation or another, remain fundamental to medical practice because they reflect human variability in health and disease.

Statistical methods for analyzing reference values used to be restricted largely to the use of means, variances, and the well-known Normal and logNormal probability distributions.[1] As problems involving reference values in clinical medicine have deepened, statistical methods applied to them have necessarily become more extensive. They can still be seen, however, as tools for analyzing the structure of human variability and, in particular, the different components of that variability contained in reference values.

We start with the conventional "reference range," defined by a pair of numbers (the reference limits) that bound the central 95 percent of a collection of values (the set of reference values) obtained from a specified group of individuals (the reference subjects). The word *central* means that 2.5 percent of the values lie above the upper limit and 2.5 percent below the lower limit. The reference subjects comprise a sample drawn from a much larger population, more or less well defined. The sampling pro-

---

[1] The normal probability distribution is deeply embedded in statistics. To avoid confusion with "normal range" or "normal" in the sense of typical or ideal, we follow the suggestion of Healy (1969b) to capitalize the first letter when referring to this distribution.

cess has seldom been statistically random, that is, following rules of probability sampling.[2]

In principle, the domain of reference ranges goes beyond the traditional "normal" range to represent data from other groups of individuals besides the healthy. For example, the distribution of thyroid-related biochemical profiles has been examined in hypo- and hyperthyroid patients (e.g., Homburger and Hewan-Lowe, 1979). However, the object of these and similar studies of biochemical analytes in sick patients has not been to produce reference ranges but to find specific values of these analytes that show optimal ability to discriminate between states of health and disease. Such cutpoints are certainly reference values, but the development of reference ranges as such is still generally confined to healthy individuals.

Credit for the concept of "reference" range belongs to Gräsbeck and Saris (1969), who, like others, were troubled by the vagueness and ambiguity of the word "normal," especially as it relates to health, another term difficult to define precisely. For example, according to one definition of the normal range in laboratory medicine, it should represent the typical or usual determinations found in active, freely functioning individuals. A more restrictive definition would have the normal range represent an ideal standard of persons demonstrably free of disease and observed under conditions that minimize physiological stress.

Gräsbeck and Saris's purpose in changing the name to reference range was to emphasize that, whichever definition the investigator preferred, the individuals forming the reference sample and the conditions under which they were observed should be described as fully as possible. Different characteristics of the reference sample (e.g., by age or sex, in health or post-treatment for a given disease), or different pre-analytical rules (e.g., patients fasting or nonfasting, lying down or sitting up),

---

[2] Notable exceptions are the Sherbrooke study of Munan et al. (1978) and the National Health and Nutrition Surveys of the U.S. National Center for Health Statistics (e.g., see Fulwood et al., 1987).

or different analytical methods could be expected to produce different reference ranges for the same biochemical analyte. An explicit description of the reference subjects and the conditions of sampling and analysis becomes then a necessary part of the definition and use of a set of reference values (Alström, 1981).

The reference range provides a guideline to the clinician or clinical chemist seeking to interpret a measurement obtained from a new patient. If possible, the user should select a reference range derived from a sample of individuals whose characteristics most closely match those of the patient. Moreover, the range should be based on an analytical method similar to the one used by the clinical laboratory that produced the new measurement. These days, especially in the United States, many reference ranges are developed by the manufacturers of analytical instruments and reagents, who then face the practical problem of making the set of reference values and description of the reference subjects available on request. More difficult to resolve is the problem of transference, that is, assuring that a reference range determined by the manufacturer will be valid in a clinical laboratory using the manufacturer's equipment. We address this problem briefly in Chapter 3. Finally, cost considerations severely limit the number of different reference ranges that can be developed for any one analyte.

The conventional reference range is a cross-sectional index derived from a collection of measurements made on many individuals, each of whom has contributed a single value. It follows that the use of such ranges is generally limited to diagnostic screening where only a single measurement of a biochemical analyte or other quantity has been obtained from the patient. Once a series of measurements over time have been obtained, the clinician will interpret any new measurement by reference to the previous observations and will no longer need a group-based range. Instead, questions then arise about the statistical (and clinical) significance of trends or sudden departures from earlier levels.

This is especially true in patients who have already undergone treatment for a diagnosed disease and are now being routinely monitored to detect recurrence or some other change of state. The diagnostic mode has changed to the patient management mode. One might argue that, conceptually, we have merely replaced one set of reference values, that derived from a group of individuals, by another set, the patient's own history of values. For that reason we have included discussion of patient-specific reference values in this book (Chapter 7). The statistical issues and methods involved are completely different from those underlying the group-based reference ranges used to aid in diagnosis.

Many statistical questions arise in connection with the derivation and use of reference ranges. For example, are the reference values homogeneous in the sense that their distribution can be properly represented by a single mathematical formula? If this appears to be the case, can we identify this distribution, and from this calculate the desired reference range? On the other hand, if the reference sample is known to contain different demographic subgroups or genetic categories, does this warrant developing separate ranges for each subgroup? If the probability distribution representing a set of reference values cannot be identified specifically, then a *nonparametric* method (i.e., a method that does not require knowledge of the form of the underlying probability distribution) must be used to derive the reference range. How do the statistical properties of a nonparametric range compare with those of a range derived from a known probability distribution? We explore these and related questions in Chapters 2 and 3.

Not surprisingly, the actual development of reference range methodology during the past half-century did not follow this rather dry sequence of questions, but was more experimental and controversial. To our knowledge, Wootton et al. (1951) were the first to name specific probability distributions in describing variations in biochemical measurements. These workers collected blood samples from 100 actively working, presumably healthy volunteers of both sexes between the ages of 18 and 50. All were fasting for at least 4 hours before sampling. Altogether, 18 analytes were tested, in either serum or whole blood, the number of observations for each analyte ranging from 50 to 100. Wootton and colleagues reported that the data for seven analytes were Normally distributed, whereas ten analytes showed logNormal distributions. The observations for one analyte, plasma globulin, were skewed to the left (negative skewness).

Although these probability distributions were mentioned and curves drawn to illustrate them, they were not fitted mathematically to the corresponding observed distributions of values. Instead, lower 1 percent and 10 percent limits and upper 90 percent and 99 percent limits were calculated by inspection of the ordered array of data for each analyte. Wootton et al.'s work was later extended by Wootton and King (1953) to 27 analytes in whole blood, serum, or plasma of which about half were reported to show Normal distributions and the remainder log-Normal or negatively skewed distributions.

During the 1950s, papers began to appear on the biochemical effects of demographic differences among reference subjects and on the importance of pre-analytical conditions such as the individual's posture and previous food intake [see Wootton (1962) for a brief review of this work]. However, the decade of the 1960s introduced a controversy considerably enlivening the study of "normal" ranges (the terminology of the time). The argument was probably one of the driving forces behind both scientific and official concern with the subject of reference ranges. We turn now to this question.

1.2 REFERENCE RANGES FROM HOSPITAL PATIENTS?

The debate seemed to revolve about a statistical method for deriving normal ranges from hospital laboratory data proposed by Pryce (1960) and supported by Hoffmann (1963). In fact, the roots of the problem lay deeper than that and are not yet entirely resolved. One issue concerned the very definition and purpose of normal ranges (see below). Further, it had become clear, particularly through the studies of Belk and Sunderman (1947) and Wootton and King (1953), that in both the United States and the United Kingdom, clinical laboratories showed wide discrepancies in their reported results from distributed split samples. It seemed proper, then, that until interlaboratory variation could be reduced to a much lower level, each hospital laboratory should develop its own set of normal ranges applicable to the population of blood samples routinely analyzed in that laboratory.

Immediately, another set of problems arose: From what source should each laboratory obtain its normal ranges? Should the hospital recruit a cadre of healthy, working volunteers from its own staff or a similar, readily available group? Would such individuals be available in sufficient numbers to produce reliable normal ranges, and, more importantly, would they adequately represent the range of demographic, occupational, and genetic characteristics seen among the populace served by the hospital? Would not the routine data that the laboratory already has in great abundance from its own patients be a better source, both in terms of numbers and representativeness? But, then, how could patient data produce a range that could legitimately be called "normal"? What is the purpose of a so-called normal range, anyway?

Pryce argued that for any analyte, the great majority of samples analyzed in the clinical laboratory were, indeed, normal, or at least representative of active, nonhospitalized individuals. As he pointed out, standards of health for persons to be sampled for normal ranges were as yet undefined. Moreover, Pryce claimed that the distribution of this major "normal" component of laboratory test data was Normal in form.[3] Therefore, he proposed that the entire cumulative distribution of results for a given analyte be plotted on Normal probability paper and a straight line fitted by eye to that portion of the distribution that appeared to plot linearly, usually the majority of observations.

---

[3] Pryce believed that moderately skewed distributions were typical of hospital data as a whole but had not found that transformation to logarithms produced Normal symmetry.

Then, he estimated the mode of the entire distribution[4] and used this to represent the mean of the Normal component. The standard deviation (SD) was then calculated from those observations that fell on the presumably "normal" side of the mode. The 95 percent normal range would then be the estimated mode ±2 SD.

Hoffmann (1963) suggested extending the eye-fitted straight line to cover the 2.5th and 97.5th percentile points, from which perpendiculars dropped to the abscissa would yield the lower and upper limits of the normal range. Since Pryce's and Hoffmann's papers, various modifications to this method have been proposed. For example, Neumann (1968) suggested estimating the uppermost point of the "normal" component of the overall distribution, replotting all data below this point as a cumulative distribution on Normal probability paper, estimating a new (lower) maximum from a new straight line fitted by eye, and repeating the cycle until no noticeable change occurs. At that point the line should be extended and the normal range calculated as Hoffmann proposed. Becktel (1970) advocated estimating both mean and standard deviation of the normal component from selected percentiles of that portion of the distribution, using formulas adapted from results by Mosteller (1946) on "order statistics" (see Chapter 2) from a Normal distribution. Still another method, taken from the statistical literature (Bhattacharya, 1967; Gindler, 1970; Oosterhuis et al., 1990) calls for the separation of laboratory data into two assumed Normal distributions, one taken to represent normal values, the other abnormal. An even more ambitious statistical procedure for separating the two distributions, allowing for skewness in each one, was proposed by Martin et al. (1975, pp. 334–351).

None of these methods has gained general acceptance, either because of unwarranted assumptions or mathematical

---

[4] Using an old formula (Doodson, 1917) for moderately skewed distributions, namely, that the mode is equal to the mean − 3(mean − median).

complexity or both. The attractive idea that any hospital or other clinical laboratory could develop its own set of reference ranges by somehow extracting a normal component of laboratory values from a mixture of patient data has not resulted in reliable methods worthy or, in some cases, even capable of routine application.

By the late 1960s reaction against the Pryce-Hoffmann methods had begun to appear in print. The most frequently cited paper, that of Amador and Hsi (1969), defined methods that derive normal ranges from routine hospital laboratory data as "indirect" procedures in contrast to "direct" estimation of normal ranges from selected groups of apparently healthy individuals. Amador and Hsi estimated means and standard deviations for six analytes (three enzymes, blood glucose, urea nitrogen, serum cholesterol) from 50–100 active working subjects, both men and women, largely hospital employees (note the similarity to the 1951 study of Wootton et al.). They compared these statistics with similar estimates using the Pryce-Hoffmann and other indirect methods applied to 500 consecutive laboratory results from adult hospital patients. Except for cholesterol, mean values based on the indirect methods were almost always higher than an upper 95 percent confidence limit for the true mean as estimated from the healthy subjects, whereas standard deviations were usually larger than the upper confidence limit for the true SD as estimated from the healthy group.[5]

Amador and Hsi cited analogous results for serum sodium, chloride, potassium, and bicarbonate concentrations obtained by Van Peenen and Lindberg (1965) and for sodium by Payne and Levell (1967), namely, estimated ranges under Pryce's or a similar procedure biased toward the abnormal region and

---

[5] Unfortunately, the confidence interval computed by Amador and Hsi for the true standard deviation depends heavily on the assumption of a Normal distribution, which was probably not satisfied for these analytes even among healthy individuals. Nevertheless, the direction of the comparisons was clear.

wider, indicating a more heterogeneous set of supposedly normal test results than was obtained from healthy subjects. Their conclusion was that physicians tended to order a given test when the patient was "suspected or known to have an abnormal test result, thereby shifting the mode toward pathologic levels," rendering unacceptable a normal range based on routine clinical laboratory data.

This conclusion was supported several years later by Reed et al. (1972) who noted that prior to 1970, the chief reason for requesting laboratory tests was to confirm clinical diagnoses or to investigate suspected abnormalities. However, at the time of their writing, it was becoming increasingly common to request fixed batteries of laboratory tests, determined, in part, by the advent of multichannel analyzers specifically designed to perform multiple determinations on a given specimen. (More recently, routine ordering of test profiles on admission has markedly declined.)

Further criticism of the use of hospital patients to derive reference ranges in health was contained in a well-known paper by Elveback et al.(1970). These authors presented data on serum calcium, phosphorus, total protein, albumin, magnesium, alkaline phosphatase, and urea from 576 active, working persons who showed "no significant abnormal findings" after biochemical, hematological, and X-ray examinations. Even among such presumably healthy individuals, all the analytes except albumin showed non-Normal distributions. Applying the Pryce-Hoffmann method to hundreds or thousands of consecutive laboratory test values on adult patients in their hospital (Mayo Clinic) during the same time period, they obtained unacceptably wide 95 percent ranges.

Nevertheless, the proposals by Pryce and Hoffmann made two important contributions, in our opinion. First, they focused attention not only on the statistical distributions of cross-sectional biochemical test data, but, more generally, on the heterogeneity of reference populations, whether hospital patients or healthy subjects. Second, they raised questions about the definition and purpose of a normal range, and, more recently, reference ranges in general.

1.3 HETEROGENEITY AMONG REFERENCE SUBJECTS

During the late 1960s and the 1970s, partly in response to the controversy surrounding the use of laboratory data from a hospital population, a number of reports appeared showing statistically significant variations in many common biochemical analytes by age, sex, and other characteristics (e.g., the use of oral contraceptives) across large samples of presumably healthy persons. In particular, we note the works of Roberts (1967), Keating et al. (1969), Werner et al. (1970), Reed et al. (1972), Wilding et al. (1972), Winkelman et al. (1973), Flynn et al. (1974, 1976), and McPherson et al. (1978).

Large, essentially unselected samples of individuals attending well-person screening centers provided the data of Wilding et al. (approximately 4800 persons) and Werner et al. (over 3000). Over 1400 specimens analyzed by Reed and co-workers were submitted by internists from four broad geographic regions of the United States. In none of these studies was control possible over the time of day at which blood specimens were drawn or the fasting or nonfasting condition of the subject. Keating et al. selected 576 healthy persons undergoing annual employment examinations or routine checkups. Roberts' sample was much smaller, including slightly under 300 blood donors from whom specimens were collected between 10 and 11:30 A.M. while subjects lay supine for 5 minutes before collection. Flynn et al. also sampled blood donors (1022) during the morning hours. Volunteers included in all of these studies were checked for general good health as well as absence of chronic disease and therapeutic drugs. Analyses were performed on multichannel autoanalyzers or single-test automated procedures.

Various methods were employed to judge the statistical significance of age–sex group differences, including regression analysis, multiple-comparison nonparametric tests, and repeated Normal deviate z-tests or Student's t-tests.[6] Many statistically significant differences among age–sex groups were found and compared with those reported in earlier studies. We shall not review these details, but shall pause briefly to consider some general effects of heterogeneous populations.

The use of a single reference range to represent subgroups of individuals with substantially different means or variances raises several problems. Two statistical consequences are (1) that the combination of such subgroups will generally produce a non-Normal distribution, and (2) that the variance of the combined distribution will be greater than the variances of the separate subgroups. This would lead to a wider reference range, less sensitive to abnormalities.

The non-Normal distribution can be dealt with either by transformation to Normal form through a change of measurement scale or by using nonparametric methods (Chapter 2). The increase in variance turns out to be surprisingly small unless the differences among subgroup means are extremely large. We discuss this more fully in Chapter 3 but illustrate the point here with data on serum albumin presented by Wilding et al. (1972).

These authors, like others, found "highly significant" decreases among both men and women in the mean values of serum albumin from the third through the eighth age decades. Results for men are shown in Table 1.1.

The average standard deviation within each age decade is computed as the square root of $\Sigma n_i s_i^2 / N$, where $N = 3717$, the total number of men. The result is 0.217. Despite the statistically highly significant decrease of mean value with age, the reduction in the average within-age standard deviation compared to the standard deviation in the combined group is only 3.4 percent: $100(0.225 - 0.217)/.225$. It is, in fact, a commmon result, discussed in greater detail by Harris and Boyd (1990) and in

---

[6] The last two methods are unreliable unless steps are taken to control the probability of false rejection of the Null hypothesis at a predetermined level (e.g., <0.05) for each application of the test.

Table 1.1 Mean and Standard Deviation (g/100 mL) of Serum Albumin in Men, by Age

Age decade (i)	Number (n_i)	Mean ($\bar{x}_i$)	Standard deviation (s_i)
20–29	96	4.41	0.20
30–39	721	4.35	0.21
40–49	1268	4.29	0.21
50–59	1112	4.24	0.22
60–69	415	4.19	0.22
70–79	105	4.13	0.30
Combined	3717	4.27	0.225

Source: Wilding et al. (1972, Table III, p. 379).

Chapter 3, that subgroups whose means are significantly different statistically show only slightly less variation within themselves than when all subgroups are lumped together. The argument that separate subgroup reference ranges would be substantially narrower than the combined range is seldom supported by the results.

There is another consequence of using a single reference range to cover heterogeneous subgroups that we believe has more serious clinical implications. In the presence of subgroup differences, a reference range that includes a central proportion (say, the central 95 percent) of the combined distribution does not include the same proportion of the subgroup distributions. For example, the combined reference range may include close to 100 percent of one subgroup distribution, whereas for another subgroup a much larger (smaller) proportion than expected of the high values but a much smaller (larger) proportion than expected of the low values are excluded. Thus, the diagnostic implications of the combined range may be misleading for the individual patient. We examine this problem in Chapter 3 where criteria for establishing separate reference ranges are considered.

1.4 PURPOSES OF REFERENCE RANGES FOR THE HEALTHY

As mentioned earlier, we believe that one of the chief contributions of the Pryce-Hoffman proposals was to focus attention on the definition and essential purpose of the reference range (then restricted to the "normal" range). Indeed, 10 years after his suggested method appeared in print, Pryce (1970) claimed that since physicians are "exclusively concerned with people seeking medical advice, and have no direct knowledge of, or concern with, those not seeking such advice," normal ranges should be derived from that population, that is, patients with varying degrees of illness.

This view has not been widely shared. For example, McCall (1966) argued on the contrary that the normal range in medical practice represents an "ideal standard," indicative of good health. He stated that "A medically useful normal range will then be the statistical normal range determined in a selected healthy population, thereby establishing a standard range against which degrees of ill health can be recognised." An observation outside this range would then reflect a nonphysiological condition that, even if not labeled as a specific disease, should be corrected, if possible. Keyser (1965) supported this purpose of the normal range, noting, as an example, that if one wished to measure the effectivess of dietary therapy in lowering serum cholesterol, the desired range of values would be that found in "the most carefully selected, healthy subjects."

This point of view, not so explicitly stated, underlies the studies of Keating et al., Roberts, and Flynn et al., in particular the practice of deriving normal ranges from blood donors. It stands apart, however, from another belief (closer to but clearly distinct from Pryce's) that the normal range should be the usual or prevailing condition in a large, relatively unselected, but active, working population. This is essentially the definition used by Werner et al. and Wilding et al. More recently (1981), Siest, chairman of the Commission on Reference Values of the French Society of Clinical Biology, has advocated the use of well-person screening programs as a source of reference values in healthy persons.

Under this viewpoint, the normal range in an elderly population would reflect common disabilities of age, just as higher cholesterol values in postmenopausal women result from declining estrogen levels. Does it necessarily follow, then, that the "normal" cholesterol level in older women and men is a desirable or even acceptable state? Epidemiological studies and the decision levels currently proposed in the effort to prevent heart disease would indicate otherwise (see Section 1.7 and Chapter 8, Section 8.4).

1.5 OFFICIAL GUIDELINES ON SELECTION AND TREATMENT OF REFERENCE SUBJECTS

The selection of reference subjects is clearly of critical importance to the eventual use of the reference values. Similarly, the treatment of reference subjects preceding and during sample collection, as well as the method of biochemical analysis used, will affect the distribution of values obtained and the validity of the reference range as a reliable guide to the clinician.

These topics have been the special concerns of committees appointed by various national societies of clinical chemistry, especially in Europe, to develop "official" guidelines for obtaining reference values. The first of these reports appeared in 1975, authored by Alström et al., who constituted the Committee on Reference Values of the Scandinavian Society for Clinical Chemistry and Clinical Physiology. This was followed by a series of reports (1979–85; earlier versions appeared during the 1970s) by the Commission on Reference Values of the French Society of Clinical Biology. Similar documents were published by the Spanish Society for Clinical Chemistry during 1983–85. Finally, the International Federation for Clinical Chemistry (IFCC), through its Expert Panel on Reference Values, published during the 1980s a series of recommendations on the topics of selection and treatment of reference subjects as well as the statistical analysis of reference values.

In a symposium volume on reference values in laboratory medicine (1981), Alström has provided an informative review of earlier versions of these various reports. In the same volume, Berg et al. described the results of an unsuccessful application of the comprehensive, but rather rigid selection rules that appeared in the 1975 report of the Scandinavian Society mentioned earlier. In another paper of this symposium, Statland and Winkel discussed pre-analytical sources of biological variation and the importance of controlling them. For an earlier, more complete review of this subject, see Statland and Winkel (1977); a book on this topic is now available (Young, 1993). Finally, we recommend a recent review by Solberg and Gräsbeck (1989), who summarize the concepts, points of view, and methods related to all these issues and provide an extensive bibliography of both scientific sources and official reports.

American societies for clinical chemistry have been slower than their European counterparts to organize formal efforts to deal with the issues of reference values although individual scientists early recognized the poorly defined nature of "normal" ranges (e.g., Benson, 1972). In particular, an editorial in *Clinical Chemistry* by Sunderman (1975) supporting the concept of reference values in contrast to "normal values" was influential in drawing the attention of American clinical chemists to the subject. The National Committee for Clinical Laboratory Standards (NCCLS) established a subcommittee on reference intervals that issued a preliminary report in early 1992.

1.6 CRITICISMS OF THE NORMAL RANGE

Leaving aside the question of definition, the normal range concept has been subjected to deeper criticisms, including the following:

1. The 95 percent (or any percent) normal range creates an unrealistic dichotomy between "normal" and "abnormal" or "health" and "disease." Concentrations of biochemical analytes form a continuous scale, and important diagnostic information

is lost when a continuous measurement is arbitrarily classified as either normal or abnormal. One mitigating factor is that the normal range is only one of many guidelines, numerical and verbal, that physicians use to evaluate the historical, physical, and laboratory data available for most patients. Nevertheless, the criticism is clearly valid, and various authors, including Healy (1969), Elveback (1972), and Weldon and Mackay (1972a) have recommended that laboratories report not only the measured value, but also the percentile of the reference population whose values lie below the measured value. This requires that the laboratory have access to the distribution of values in the reference population. Unfortunately, these data have generally not been available to the great majority of clinical laboratories, which depend on ranges provided by the manufacturers of analytical procedures and reagents used in the laboratory.

2. Multiple normal ranges reported for batteries of tests create a special dilemma (Schoen and Brooks, 1970; Sunderman, 1970; Reed, 1970; Sackett, 1973; Healy, 1979). The probability that an individual free of disease will show all test values within their respective ranges gets smaller as the number of tests increase. Assuming independent test results, the probability that all will lie within their p percent (e.g., 95 percent) normal ranges is p^k, where k is the number of tests. Therefore, the probability that at least one will show a falsely abnormal result is $1 - p^k$, equal to about 60 percent for $p = 0.95$ and a battery of ten tests. The danger of wasted time, effort, and money spent in following up false-positive results becomes a serious concern.

A theoretical solution to this problem lies in widening the normal range for each analyte so that the overall probability of one false positive out of n tests remains at 0.95. This is not practical because the number of tests carried out on a single specimen will vary greatly. More importantly, widening each range will only render it even more insensitive than normal ranges already are to values observed in the presence of disease.

Weldon and Mackay (1972b) pointed out that tests that are independent in health are often correlated in the diseased state, reflecting different aspects of the same pathological condition.

They gave the example of alkaline phosphatase and serum bilirubin in obstruction of the common bile duct. Indeed, laboratories provide, and clinicians are accustomed to ordering, panels of selected tests that together indicate the state of a particular organ system, helping the physician determine the correct diagnosis among a set of competing possibilities.

In these situations, multivariate reference regions or indexes in different disease states, taking into account the correlations between pairs of tests, would be more reliable diagnostic aids than multiple univariate ranges. This topic is discussed in Chapter 4.

3.   A more fundamental criticism has been leveled against normal ranges by many writers on the subject [an early source is Murphy and Abbey (1967)]. This is that a test measurement cannot be properly evaluated unless the distributions of such measurements in specific disease states are also available. If the distribution of test values under a diseased state overlaps the distribution in healthy persons, the best "discrimination point" (Sunderman, 1975) for distinguishing the two alternatives will rarely be the upper (or lower) limit of the standard normal range. Rather, it will depend on the amount of overlap, the prevalence of the disease, and the costs (physical, social, economic, etc.) of failing to detect a patient with the disease or, conversely, of treating a patient falsely believed to have the disease.

In practice, the cost of determining the distributions of selected analytes in specific disease states may be very high, requiring painstaking search through medical records. Moreover, such distributions will often have their own unique characteristics, not only for different age–sex groups, but also for different stages of the disease. It is not surprising, therefore, given these difficulties, and the innate conservatism of medical practice, that the reference range in healthy persons has proved to be such a durable concept despite the drawbacks described earlier. For example, it is still the basis for the great majority of "decision levels" listed in a recent text (Statland, 1987). The reference range in healthy persons remains a guideline widely used by physicians and is one of the first statistical properties investigated whenever a new biochemical test is reported. However, competing ideas are gaining increasing attention in clinical practice.

1.7 DECISION LEVELS AND PATIENT MONITORING

In one important area of medical and public health concern, the detection and treatment of coronary heart disease, the reference range as a diagnostic aid has been abandoned and quite independent decision levels have been developed and widely accepted among clinicians. These critical values (sometimes called "threshold" values) have been derived from prospective epidemiological studies directly relating the risk of coronary heart disease to measured concentrations of total cholesterol (see Figure 1.1).

From these data, the Report of the National Cholesterol Education Program (NCEP) Expert Panel (1988) of the National Heart and Blood Institute established the following criteria for interpreting serum total cholesterol values: Levels below 200 mg/dL are classified as "desirable blood cholesterol," those 200–239 mg/dL as "borderline-high cholesterol," and those 240 mg/dL and above as "high blood cholesterol." These are now the operative reference values for serum cholesterol. The Report of the NCEP noted that 240 mg/dL corresponds to the 75th percentile for the adult U.S. population, but clearly it was the change in risk of coronary heart disease, not the distribution of cholesterol in the total population (nor any reference range derived from that distribution), that determined the selection of 240 mg/dL as a critical point.

The clinical use of specified cutpoints as decision levels for medical action (even when such cutpoints are the upper or lower limits of the standard reference range) raises a set of statistical issues quite separate from the problem of the overlapping distributions of analyte values in healthy and diseased populations. For example, new definitions of sensitivity and

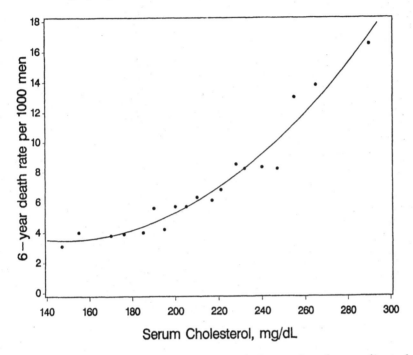

Fig. 1.1 Relationship of initial serum cholesterol and age-adjusted rate of coronary heart disease during average follow-up period of 6 years in men 35–57 years of age at initial visit. (From Report of the National Cholesterol Education Program Expert Panel, 1988.)

specificity are required, and the roles of analytical bias and imprecision as related to inherent biological variation are changed. We explore these statistical questions in Chapter 8.

In still another clinical context, the reference range has begun to give way. As noted in the Preface, the work of clinical laboratories has become increasingly devoted to the management rather than the diagnosis of patients' illnesses. It follows that, more and more, repeated measurements over time are available on specific analytes in individual patients. Here, as mentioned earlier, the traditional cross-sectional reference range offers little help in evaluating the patient's status. Instead, clinicians compare a current measurement with the patient's own history of test values. Objective, statistical methods for reaching decisions from serial records, even short series, on the same patient are appearing more often, although mainly in clinical research studies rather than general practice. We describe some methods for this purpose in Chapter 7.

2

CALCULATING REFERENCE LIMITS

2.1 INTRODUCTION

In this and the following chapter, we discuss some special statistical topics of importance to reference ranges. These include (1) statistical methods for calculating reference ranges, (2) sample size (the number of reference subjects in study), (3) criteria for deciding whether to develop separate reference ranges for subgroups in the population, (4) the treatment of outlying observations, and (5) the transference of reference ranges. This chapter is devoted to the first of these topics.

By convention, we seek to estimate the central 95 percent reference range: specifically, the percentiles $\zeta_{0.025}$ and $\zeta_{0.975}$, defined as those values such that exactly 2.5 percent of the population of values are less than or equal to the former, and 97.5 percent of the population are less than or equal to the latter.

There are many methods described in the literature for estimating percentiles from a collection of measurements. These divide into the broad categories of parametric and nonparametric procedures. For our purposes, the class of parametric methods consists of various "Normalizing" transformations, formulas for converting the original measurements of the analyte to a scale on which the distribution of values will conform to the Normal model. This allows estimation of $\zeta_{0.025}$ and $\zeta_{0.975}$ by simply adding and subtracting from the mean of the transformed values 1.96 times the standard deviation of those values. There are good grounds in statistical theory for deriving estimates from a Normal distribution. Unfortunately, the process of finding the scale on which the observations are Normally distributed can be rather complicated.

The nonparametric process is generally simpler because it rests on no particular mathematical model of the distribution of values in the population from which the reference sample has been drawn. Like a parametric procedure, it does assume that there exists an underlying homogeneous probability distribution, even if not mathematically identified. Both parametric and nonparametric estimates of extreme percentiles are sensitive to observations far removed from the main body of results. For reasons known or unknown, these may be contaminants, originating from a different distribution than the rest of the reference set and compromising the reliability of reference limits computed from the entire set. Further discussion of the problem of outliers is deferred until Chapter 3.

There is also another concern, the question of the statistical randomness of the sampling procedure that led to the selection of reference subjects. As mentioned in Chapter 1, very few studies to derive reference values for healthy individuals can claim to have collected a statistically random sample of healthy subjects from some predefined population, that is, to have followed a sampling process that provided every member of the population an equal opportunity to be part of the sample.[1] The large body of statistical theory that deals with inferring population parameters (means, variances, percentiles, etc.) from sample statistics rests on the assumption that the sample has been drawn by a random process. On the other hand, the absence of strictly random sampling does not necessarily preclude the validity of estimates based on the observed sample of measurements. We simply hope that the sample is reasonably representative of the desired population, and that whatever unknown characteristics make it imperfectly representative do not seriously bias the estimates obtained from the sample. Whether or not this is merely a pious hope can be judged to some extent by comparison with estimates from other studies of the same or apparently similar populations.

---

[1] To provide some degree of assurance that the sample includes only healthy persons, the use of questionnaires and various possible exclusion criteria has been recommended (see Chapter 1). These devices help define the population but do not affect the randomness of the sampling.

2.2 NONPARAMETRIC ESTIMATION

2.2.1 The Quantile Estimator

We turn first to nonparametric methods of estimating $\zeta_{0.025}$ and $\zeta_{0.975}$. These methods involve ordering the n measurements by size and then assigning them ranks in sequence from 1, the smallest, to n, the largest. The ordered observations are called *order statistics*, denoted by $x_{(1)}, x_{(2)}, \ldots x_{(r)}, \ldots, x_{(n)}$. The simplest nonparametric procedure estimates $\zeta_{0.025}$ as the observation with rank $r = 0.025 \, (n + 1)$, usually denoted by $Q_{0.025}$, the 2.5 percent sample quantile. The upper reference limit, estimating $\zeta_{0.975}$, is the observation with rank $r = 0.975 \, (n + 1)$, or $Q_{0.975}$. These values of r will usually not be integers, so the quantiles are obtained by linear interpolation between the order statistics with integer ranks on either side.

2.2.2 Confidence Limits Based on the Quantile Estimator

These sample quantiles are called *point* estimates of the corresponding percentiles $\zeta_{0.025}$ and $\zeta_{0.975}$. Other examples of point estimates are the sample mean $\bar{x}$ and standard deviation s, which estimate the mean μ and standard deviation σ of the population of values from which the sample was drawn. Point estimates provide convenient summaries of the observations and are used so frequently as merely descriptive statistics that one tends to forget their role as estimators of population parameters. Another class of estimates, confidence intervals, are in fact more useful because they carry information about the reliability of point estimates.

A confidence interval estimate of a population parameter is a range of values computed from the observed data but intended to include the value of the parameter. We realize that a second confidence interval, computed from another random sample of the same size, would undoubtedly be different from the first. Therefore, included in the concept of a confidence interval estimate is a probability $(1 - \alpha)$ called the *level of confi-*

dence that $100(1 - \alpha)$ percent of such confidence intervals computed from a large number of random samples of the same size will contain the value of the parameter. The probability $(1 - \alpha)$ is commonly set at some high value like 0.90, or 0.95, or 0.99. The higher the confidence level, the wider the interval. If $(1 - \alpha)$ is set too high (α too small), the resulting interval may be so wide as to be practically useless as an estimator. If this result occurs for a reasonable value of α (0.1, for example), the sample size is too small to serve the desired purpose, and the corresponding point estimate is unreliable.

Like a point estimate, the confidence interval presumes that the observed values may be considered a random, or at least representative, sample of the population. Even if we are not entirely satisfied on this point, the confidence interval serves at least two useful purposes. First, it provides indirectly a quantitative measure of the variability of the corresponding point estimate. Second, its width narrows as the sample size increases, giving the investigator an idea of the improved precision that would be obtained if the estimate were based on a larger sample.

Confidence interval estimates of $\zeta_{0.025}$ and $\zeta_{0.975}$ may, like the point estimates $Q_{0.025}$ and $Q_{0.975}$, be expressed in terms of the sample order statistics. Let $x_{(r)}$ and $x_{(s)}$ be the rth and sth order statistics, the sample values whose ranks are r and s, respectively. We wish to find those values of r and s for which $x_{(r)}$ and $x_{(s)}$ provide a confidence interval for ζ_p (e.g., $\zeta_{0.025}$ or $\zeta_{0.975}$). The lower limit $x_{(r)}$ is found by noting that, using the binomial distribution, the probability that $x_{(r)}$ is less than or equal to ζ_p is

$$\Pr(x_{(r)} \leq \zeta_p) = \sum_{i=r}^{n} \binom{n}{i} p^i(1 - p)^{n-i},$$

where $\binom{n}{i}$ represents the number of combinations of n objects taken i at a time. Similarly, the probability that $x_{(s)}$ is greater than or equal to ζ_p is

$$\Pr(x_{(s)} \geq \zeta_p) = \sum_{i=0}^{s-1} \binom{n}{i} p^i (1 - p)^{n-i}$$

Then,[2]

$$\Pr(x_{(r)} \leq \zeta_p \leq x_{(s)}) = \Pr(x_{(s)} \geq \zeta_p) - \Pr(x_{(r)} > \zeta_p)$$

$$= \sum_{i=0}^{s-1} \binom{n}{i} p^i (1 - p)^{n-i} - \sum_{i=0}^{r-1} \binom{n}{i} p^i (1 - p)^{n-i}$$

$$= \sum_{i=r}^{s-1} \binom{n}{i} p^i (1 - p)^{n-i}.$$

Thus, $x_{(r)}$ and $x_{(s)}$ will be the bounds of a $100(1 - \alpha)$ percent confidence interval for ζ_p if

$$\sum_{i=r}^{s-1} \binom{n}{i} p^i (1 - p)^{n-i} \geq 1 - \alpha. \tag{2.1}$$

In practice, s is chosen equal to $n - r + 1$. Equation (2.1) is valid for any continuous distribution of values in the population. The summation on the left-hand side may be written as the difference between two cumulative binomial distributions (the first summing from r to n and the second from s to n) and may be calculated from the incomplete beta distribution.[3] However,

---

[2] The following derivation, taken from Rohatgi (1984, p. 499), assumes that the distribution of x is continuous.

[3] The incomplete beta distribution $B(k, n - k)$, where k and n are integers, is

$$n!/(k - 1)!(n - k)! \int_0^p t^{k-1} (1 - t)^{n-k} \, dt, \qquad (0 < p < 1),$$

and is equal to

$$\sum_{i=k}^{n} \binom{n}{i} p^i (1 - p)^{n-i}.$$

some trial and error is needed to satisfy the inequality in Equation (2.1). Table 2.1, based on this equation and taken from Reed et al. (1971), lists the ranks of the ordered observations that provide 90 percent confidence intervals for $\zeta_{0.025}$ and $\zeta_{0.975}$ from samples in the size range 120–369.

For example, with 300 subjects, the 90 percent confidence interval for $\zeta_{0.025}$ is $x_{(3)} - x_{(13)}$, while the 90 percent confidence interval for $\zeta_{0.975}$ is $x_{(288)} - x_{(298)}$. As indicated in the table, the minimum number of subjects (n) for which exact nonparametric

Table 2.1 Nonparametric 90 Percent Confidence Intervals for Reference Limits[a]

No. of samples, n		Rank	
From	To	r	s
120	131	1	7
132	159	1	8
160	187	1	9
188	189	1	10
190	216	2	10
217	246	2	11
247	251	2	12
252	276	3	12
277	307	3	13
308	310	3	14
311	338	4	14
339	366	4	15
367	369	5	15

Source: Reed et al. (1971), Table 3, p. 281.
[a] The rth lowest sample values = lower limit of 90 percent confidence interval for $\zeta_{0.025}$ in sampled population; the sth lowest sample value = upper limit of 90 percent confidence interval for $\zeta_{0.025}$ in sampled population. To obtain ranks corresponding to a 90 percent confidence interval for $\zeta_{0.975}$, subtract the values given for r and s from $n + 1$.

90 percent confidence intervals can be obtained for these percentiles is 120. For $n < 120$, the lower limit of the 90 percent confidence interval for $\zeta_{0.025}$ can be defined only as less than the smallest observation, while the upper limit of the 90 percent confidence interval for $\zeta_{0.975}$ can be defined only as greater than the largest observation.

For large sample sizes, there exists a more readily available, if approximate, nonparametric $100(1 - \alpha)$ percent confidence interval for ζ_p. This is given by the order statistics $x_{(r)}$, $x_{(s)}$, where r is the largest integer less than or equal to $np + \frac{1}{2} - z_{\alpha/2}\sqrt{np(1 - p)}$, s is the smallest integer greater than or equal to $np + \frac{1}{2} + z_{\alpha/2}\sqrt{np(1 - p)}$; and $z_{\alpha/2}$ is the standard Normal deviate, cutting off the upper $(100\ \alpha/2)$ percent of the standard Normal curve (e.g., Rohatgi, 1984, p. 617). This large-sample result is obtained by using the Normal approximation to the binomial. The addition of $\frac{1}{2}$ is a (conservative) correction to compensate for substituting a continuous for a discrete distribution. Using this approximate, but simpler, procedure when $p = 0.025$ or 0.975, the smallest value of n that will produce specific values for the 90 percent lower confidence limit for $\zeta_{.025}$ and the 90 percent upper confidence limit for $\zeta_{0.975}$ is $n = 143$.

2.2.3 Example

We apply these nonparametric methods to a set of values of alanine aminotransferase (ALT) measured in serum samples from 240 medical students (120 men, 120 women) at the University of Virginia during 1987 and 1988. The ordered observations are listed in the Appendix and grouped as a histogram in Figure 2.1.

The quantile estimates of $\zeta_{0.025}$ and $\zeta_{0.975}$ are, respectively, those observations with ranks $r = 0.025(241) = 6.025 \approx 6$, and $s = 0.975(241) = 234.975 \approx 235$. The estimates are $Q_{0.025} = 8$ U/L (international units per liter) and $Q_{0.975} = 54$ U/L. Ninety percent confidence limits for $\zeta_{0.025}$ are given by the order statistics $x_{(r)}$ and $x_{(s)}$, where r is the largest integer less than or equal to $240(0.025) + \frac{1}{2} - 1.645[(240(0.025)(0.975)]^{1/2} = 6.5 - 3.98$

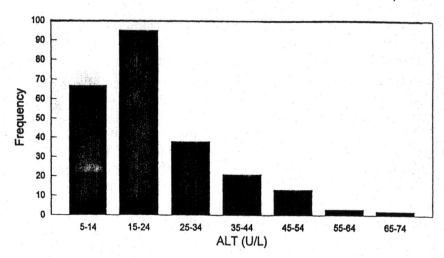

Fig. 2.1 Distribution of ALT measurements in 240 medical students.

(or $r = 2$), and s is the smallest integer greater than $6.5 + 3.98$ (or $s = 11$). Referring to the ordered observations, the desired confidence interval for $\zeta_{0.025}$ is 6–9 U/L. Similarly, 90 percent confidence limits for $\zeta_{0.975}$ are given by $x_{(r)}$ and $x_{(s)}$, where r is the largest integer less than $240(0.975) + \frac{1}{2} - 1.645 \times [(240(0.975)(0.025)]^{1/2} = 234.5 - 3.98$ (or $r = 230$) and s is the smallest integer greater than $234.5 + 3.98$ (or $s = 239$). The desired confidence interval for $\zeta_{0.975}$ is 49–65 U/L.

2.3 EFFICIENCY OF THE QUANTILE ESTIMATOR

Clearly, these nonparametric procedures for obtaining point and interval estimates for population percentiles are not difficult. For this reason and their applicability to all distributions, they are frequently used to derive reference ranges in laboratory medicine. In particular, their support by statisticians for this purpose goes back to well-known papers by Herrera (1958), Mainland (1971), and Reed et al. (1971). Apart from sensitivity to outliers, the main problem is the large sampling variation associated with quantiles in the "tails" (i.e., the extreme regions) of a set of observed reference values. As a consequence, confidence intervals for the upper reference limit may be rather wide. In the preceding example, this confidence interval was 35 percent of the entire reference range (16/46).

This kind of result can be predicted from the large-sample formula for the variance of a sample quantile,

$$V(Q_p) = p(1 - p)/(nf_p^2), \tag{2.2}$$

where f_p is the ordinate at the pth percentile of the mathematical function that represents the distribution of values in the population.

Most well-behaved distribution functions have "high contact" (i.e., gradually approach zero frequency) at one or the other, or both, tails of the distribution. For example, the Normal probability function has high contact for both large and small values relative to the mean, as indicated by its bell-shaped appearance. Skewed distributions may approach zero frequency abruptly on one side, but gradually on the other. For the large majority of analytes measured in clinical laboratories, the distributions of values are continuous curves gradually approaching the x-axis on one (usually the higher) or both ends of the distribution. This implies that for values of p close to zero or to unity, or both, f_p is close to zero. It follows from Equation (2.2) that the variances of quantiles $Q_{0.025}$ and, especially, $Q_{0.975}$ are likely to be large, even for large sample sizes.

For example, suppose the distribution of values in the population is Normal with mean μ and standard deviation σ. Then the ordinate of the distribution at any value x is given by $f(x) = [1/\sigma(2\pi)^{1/2}] \exp -\frac{1}{2}[(x - \mu)/\sigma]^2$. At $\zeta_{0.5}$, the median, the ordinate is $1/\sigma(2\pi)^{1/2}$. But at $\zeta_{0.975} = \mu + 1.96\sigma$, the ordinate is $[(1/\sigma(2\pi)^{1/2}] \exp(-1.92)$. Therefore, from Equation (2.2), the ratio of the variance of $Q_{0.975}$ to the variance of $Q_{0.5}$ is 0.0975 $\exp(3.84)$, or 4.54. In other words, if the distribution of values in the population is Normal, the variance of $Q_{0.975}$ as an estimator of $\zeta_{0.975}$ is 4.54 times the variance of the sample median as an estimator of the population median.

This is not the variance ratio we are interested in, however. If we knew beforehand that the distribution was Normal, we would not use the nonparametric estimate $Q_{0.975}$ to estimate the upper limit of the central 95 percent reference range but, rather, the parametric estimator $\bar{x} + 1.96s$, where $\bar{x}$ is the mean and s the standard deviation of the sample of reference values.[4] How does the variance of this parametric estimator compare with the variance of $Q_{0.975}$ when the underlying distribution is Gaussian? For large samples, the former variance [see Elveback and Taylor (1969)] is approximately $\sigma^2/n + (1.96)^2\sigma^2/2n$, or 2.92 σ^2/n. The latter variance is $(0.025)(0.975)2\pi(\sigma^2/n) \exp(3.84)$, or $7.13\sigma^2/n$. Thus, for large samples (say, $n > 100$) from a Normal distribution, the quantile estimator carries a variance 2.44 times that of the parametric estimator. In statistical terms, the *relative efficiency* of $Q_{0.975}$ under these conditions is only 41 percent (100/2.44). Another way of stating this relation is that when sampling from a Normal distribution to estimate $\zeta_{0.975}$, the quantile estimator would have to be based on 244 observations to achieve the same precision (in terms of variance or standard deviation) as the parametric estimator based on 100 observations.

Of course, the reason for selecting a nonparametric estimator is that we do not know the mathematical form of the distribution of values in the population and are unwilling to assume a specific distribution function, Normal or any other. If the distribution is not Normal, the parametric estimator given above will be biased, perhaps seriously so, while the quantile

---

[4] Strictly speaking, the estimator $\bar{x} + z_p s$ is not the best estimator of ζ_p in a Normal distribution. The minimum variance unbiased estimator in this case is $\bar{x} + (z_p/K_n)s$, where $K_n = [2/(n - 1)]^{1/2}\Gamma(n/2)/\Gamma[(n - 1)/2]$. For n even, $\Gamma(n/2) = (n/2 - 1)(n/2 - 2) \ldots (1)$; for n odd, $\Gamma(n/2) = (n/2 - 1)(n/2 - 2) \ldots (3/2)(1/2)(\pi^{1/2})$. For $n > 60$, K_n is so close to unity that including it increases z_p by less than 0.01. Therefore, we have neglected this factor in calculating the Normal distribution estimator of ζ_p.

estimator Q_p remains unbiased. Its average value over many samples from the population will equal ζ_p. Nevertheless, we may ask whether more precise as well as unbiased nonparametric estimators of reference limits can be obtained. The answer is yes, but the gain in precision is not great.

2.4 MORE PRECISE NONPARAMETRIC ESTIMATES

Proposals to improve the efficiency of nonparametric quantile estimators of ζ_p have followed two general paths: (1) the *kernel* method, whereby a weighting function called a kernel is applied to all or some of the quantiles in the sample to produce a weighted average quantile as the new estimator; (2) the *spline* method, whereby the entire observed cumulative distribution of values is replaced by a series of cubic polynomial segments joined together to produce a smooth curve. The quantile estimator is then determined from this smoothed representation of the cumulative distribution.

We shall discuss here only the kernel method.[5] Recently, Sheather and Marron (1990) have provided a general theoretical framework for kernel-based quantile estimators and have compared various kernel methods through Monte Carlo simulation

---

[5] We omit the spline method for several reasons: (1) applying this method to empirical data whose cumulative distribution shows considerable irregularity (as is common with cross-sectional reference data in laboratory medicine) requires a high degree of statistical judgment, experience, and computing expertise to determine the most appropriate smoothing parameters for different portions of the cumulative distribution; (2) in the one reported study (Shultz et al., 1985) where spline and kernel procedures have been compared on distributions modeled after laboratory data, the former seems generally to have produced no more precise estimates than the latter; (3) one kernel procedure that appears to be a practical candidate for application to such data is equivalent to *bootstrapping*, an alternative estimation procedure that has the advantage of providing a direct estimate of the standard error of the weighted quantile.

studies. In our opinion, the most promising kernel procedure for estimating percentiles has been proposed by Harrell and Davis (1982).

Reasoning from the formula for the expected value of the ith order statistic, these authors estimate ζ_p by a weighted average of all the observed order statistics, expressible as

$$\hat{\zeta}_p = \sum_{i=1}^{n} W_{n,i}(p)x_{(i)} \tag{2.3}$$

where the weight function (or kernel) is given by the difference between two incomplete beta functions, and $\sum_{i=1}^{n} W_{n,i}(p) = 1$. For samples of at least 100 observations, this estimator will be essentially unbiased and Normally distributed. Programs for computing the weights are available in many statistical programming systems (e.g., the Probbeta function in SAS, the Statistical Analysis System). Applying this program to the ALT data examined earlier, we estimated $\xi_{0.975}$ at 53.8 U/L, very close to the sample quantile $Q_{0.975} = 54$ U/L.

A kernel estimator is a smoothing device whereby the estimate at a chosen point (e.g., a specified percentile of the population of values) is a weighted average of all the values observed in a random sample. The heaviest weights are applied to observations in the vicinity of the chosen point. Thus, each estimate is influenced by other estimates in its neighborhood, moderating the effects of irregularities in the data. For example, the weights in Equation (2.3) for $n = 240$ and $p = 0.95$ are less than 10^{-5} for order statistics less than $x_{(209)}$, that is, for observations below $Q_{0.87}$. From this point, they rise steadily to a maximum value of 0.121 at $Q_{0.95}$, then drop to below 10^{-5} again at $x_{(239)}$, or $Q_{0.992}$.

With modern computing equipment and access to a program like the SAS Probbeta routine, the Harrell-Davis formula may be applied speedily to many percentiles of the population. Results may then be smoothed by eye or curve fitting to provide the guide called for by Elveback (1972) and others (see Section 1.6) that would allow the clinician to estimate the exact percentile corresponding to a measurement of the analyte in a new patient. Figure 2.2 shows such a curve, drawn by eye, through

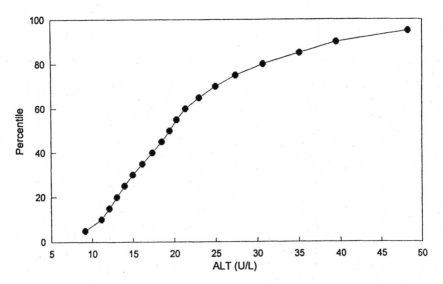

Fig. 2.2 Percentiles of ALT estimated by Harrell-Davis formula.

estimated percentiles of ALT from $p = 0.05$ to $p = 0.95$ by steps of 0.05.

Kernel estimators, expressed in more general form than Equation (2.3), have in recent years become the subject of much statistical research on nonparametric estimation of distribution functions. In Chapter 5, we mention a specific application to estimating reference percentiles dependent on time (usually age) or any covariate of interest.

Harrell and Davis compared the variance of their kernel estimator with the variance of the sample quantile from 1000 random samples generated from a variety of distributions (including Normal-like, exponential-like, and a medium-tailed asymmetric distribution), for values of n ranging from 6 to 60, and p values from 0.05 to 0.95.[6] Results varied somewhat with

---

[6] These variances are called *mean square errors* (or MSEs) because they involve squared differences from known quantities, in this case the population quantiles of different simulated distributions. Standard deviations computed under the same circumstances are called *root mean square errors*, or RMSEs.

distribution and p, but at the highest sample size, the ratio of variances for extreme values of p was never lower than 0.8, implying a 20 percent improvement in efficiency, at best. This indicates that the relative efficiency of the Harrell-Davis estimator compared to the Normal estimator is still no better than about 51 percent [100/(2.44 × 0.8)] *when the population is Normally distributed* (but see later discussion).

Schulz et al. (1985) compared the Harrell-Davis estimator with the direct sample quantile method for a number of symmetric and asymmetric distribution forms for which the true 0.025 and 0.975 percentiles could be determined. They prepared 1000 sets of 119 randomly generated observations from each distribution, calculated the estimates of $\zeta_{0.025}$ and $\zeta_{0.975}$ using both methods, and computed standard deviations for each. The ratio of the variance of the weighted quantiles estimator to that of the conventional estimator varied from .72 to .90 for the different distributions and the two values of ζ_p, thus essentially confirming the findings of Harrell and Davis. Results appeared independent of the degree of asymmetry in the underlying distribution. We refer to this study again in Section 2.5.1 in connection with transforms to convert observed distributions to Normal form.

As we mentioned earlier, the Harrell-Davis estimator expressed in the weighted quantile form is quite feasible for routine use given present-day computers and the required program. Moreover, this estimator has been shown by Sheather and Marron (1992) and others to be equal to the expected value obtained using the highly practical data sampling technique called *bootstrapping*. Bootstrapping is a computer-intensive procedure developed by Efron (1979, 1982) that has proved to be a way of obtaining efficient, asymptotically unbiased point estimates and confidence intervals. Under this method, the complete set of n observations is sampled repeatedly, each resample built up by n sequential random selections with replacement. Thus, any resample may include the same observation more than once or, perhaps, not at all. Customarily, at least 500 bootstrap resamples are obtained, and the desired estimate (in this case, the sample quantile) is calculated from each resample. The mean and variance of the estimate and a confidence interval for the parameter being estimated may then be determined from the collection of resamples. The mean quantile over a large number of resamples should be very close to if not identical with the value obtained by applying the Harrell-Davis formula, Equation (2.3), to the original sample. A $100(1 - \alpha)$ percent confidence interval for $\zeta_{0.975}$ is given by mean $Q_{0.975} \pm z_{\alpha/2}$ (SD_Q), where (SD_Q) is the standard deviation of the resample quantiles $Q_{0.975}$. A significant advantage of the bootstrapping procedure over the weighted quantile formula is that it provides both the estimate and its standard error.

Using a random number generator in the SAS programming system, we have applied bootstrapping to the ALT data. After 500 resamples, the mean value of $Q_{0.975}$, for example, was 53.25 U/L with standard deviation 2.97, leading to a 90 percent confidence interval of $53.25 \pm 1.645 (2.97)$, or $48.4 - 58.1$ U/L for $\xi_{0.975}$. This is substantially narrower than the corresponding interval, $49 - 65$, using the sample quantile estimator, because of a much decreased value for the upper confidence limit. In Section 2.5.4, we present additional examples of the increased efficiency of the bootstrapped Harrell-Davis method compared to the sample quantile estimate. At this point, however, we turn from nonparametric to parametric estimates of reference limits.

2.5 PARAMETRIC ESTIMATION: TRANSFORMATIONS TO NORMAL FORM

2.5.1 Methods from the Clinical Chemistry Literature

As noted earlier, the parametric estimator of ζ_p for large samples from a Normal distribution is $\bar{x} + z_p s$, where z_p is the standard Normal deviate such that the area under the Normal distribution ($\mu = 0$, $\sigma = 1$) from $-\infty$ to z_p is equal to p. If the "true" distribution of reference values for an analyte is not Normal, this estimator can be seriously biased, especially for extreme percentiles, even to the point of producing negative estimates. As Elveback (1970) pointed out, most analytes measured in clinical laboratories are not Normally distributed, usually because they are bounded at the low end by zero or some small positive number but can extend relatively far out on the high side. Yet it was not uncommon in earlier days for 95 percent reference limits for any analyte to be set at "the mean plus or minus two standard deviations" regardless of the asymmetry or other non-Normal attributes of the distribution.

This situation was recognized and roundly criticized during the post–World War II years by many in the clinical laboratory field [e.g., Henry (1960) and references cited therein]. The recommended solution was to transform distributions skewed to the right (as most clinical analytes appeared to be) to the logarithmic scale, estimate the desired 95 percent reference limits on this scale and then back-transform to the original units.

Studies of reference ranges have found that the simple log transformation did not always convert skewed distributions to Normal or approximately Normal form. For example, Flynn et al. (1974) noted that adding a constant (C) to the measured values before taking logs often yielded a distribution more closely approximating Normal form. These authors appear to have determined the appropriate value of C iteratively for any particular analyte, seeking to reduce to zero the coefficients of skewness and kurtosis in the transformed distribution. In Section 2.5.2, we consider the maximum likelihood estimate of C in the transform $\log(x + C)$.

The sample coefficient of skewness, usually denoted by g_1, is the ratio of the third moment about the mean (the average of cubed differences between each observation and the sample mean) to the cube of the standard deviation. For any symmetrical distribution, in particular the Normal, the expected value of g_1 is zero. For distributions skewed to the right (left), the value of g_1 is positive (negative). For large samples of size n from a Normal distribution, the sampling variance of g_1 is approximately $6/n$.

The sample coefficient of kurtosis is the ratio of the fourth moment about the mean (the average of the fourth power of differences between each observation and the sample mean) to the fourth power of the standard deviation (or the square of the variance), minus 3. This index, commonly denoted g_2, is, like g_1, a dimensionless number. The reason for subtracting 3 is that for the Normal distribution, the expected value of the ratio of the fourth moment to the square of the variance is 3, so that an effective Normalizing transformation should reduce both g_1 and g_2 to zero, within sampling variation. The coefficient of kurtosis places heavy weight on observations far from the mean. For distributions more peaked than the Normal (i.e., more closely drawn in about the mean), g_2 will be be positive; conversely, for distributions more spread out with heavier representation in shoulders than the Normal, g_2 will be negative. For large samples from a Normal distribution, the sampling variance of g_2 is approximately $24/n$.

Harris and DeMets (1972a) attempted to develop a statistical rationale for selecting particular transformations to convert non-Normal distributions of clinical reference data to Normal form. The variation in cross-sectional data arises from two basic sources: between-person biological differences and within-person variation. The latter includes variation over time in the actual concentrations of an analyte within the blood or other body fluid plus variable error due to imprecision or random bias in the analytical procedure used to measure the concentration. When the data represent measurements taken over a considerable period of time (as, for example, in the case of blood donors, where months may be required to collect data from a large sample of reference subjects), longer-term sources of analytical imprecision and bias may contribute significantly.

Between-person variation is represented by the variance of the actual (or "true") concentrations among the sampled individuals at the time each is measured. If μ_i is the true value in the ith individual, then Var μ_i denotes this variance. The variance of biological changes within the ith individual plus the variance of analytical inaccuracies in measurement may be subsumed in the term σ_i^2. Harris and DeMets showed how the skewness and kurtosis of a cross-sectional distribution of observations can be expressed as a function of these quantities. Although these shape characteristics are primarily governed by the skewness and kurtosis of the distribution of true values μ_i, the covariance of μ_i and σ_i^2 contributes to the skewness of the cross-sectional distribution, while both Var σ_i^2 (the variation of within-person variance from one individual to another) and the covariance of μ_i^2 and σ_i^2 add to the kurtosis. The covariance of μ_i and σ_i^2 will be positive when, for example, the inaccuracy of measurement or the time-to-time variability within an individual increases as the actual concentration level increases. This may help to explain the positive skewness often seen in the distributions of biochemical analytes.

Unfortunately, it is not possible mathematically to "deconstruct" an observed cross-sectional distribution into the separate contributions of these biological and analytical components of variance. However, based on their demonstration of the effects of Var σ_i^2 and covariance (μ_i, σ_i^2) on the skewness and kurtosis of such a distribution, Harris and DeMets (1972b) were led to propose a two-stage system of normalizing transformations to stabilize σ_i^2 and thereby remove a possibly major contribution to both skewness and kurtosis. Eliminating the variation in σ_i^2 associated with variation in μ_i would help decrease or remove skewness. This would reduce but not remove kurtosis; the second stage was intended to complete the task by eliminating residual variation in σ_i^2 independent of variation in μ_i.

Relationships between mean and variance in biological data have often been approximated (e.g., Taylor, 1961) by the power law $\sigma^2 = k\mu^m$, where k and m are adjustable constants and m lies between 0 and 2. As the British statistician M. S. Bartlett pointed out many years ago (1947), statistical theory predicts that when the power law holds, the new variable $z = x^{1-(m/2)}$ will show approximately constant variance, independent of μ. For $m = 1$, the square root transformation is appropriate, and for $m = 2$, the logarithmic. Harris and DeMets suggested these and the extended transform $\log(x + C)$ as possible first-stage transforms. To remove any residual non-Normal kurtosis, they proposed, following Johnson (1959), the inverse hyperbolic sine function $z_i' = \delta \sinh^{-1}(z_i/\lambda)$, where z_i ($i = 1, \ldots, n$) is the result of the first-stage transformation, standardized by subtracting its mean and dividing by its standard deviation.[7]

One drawback of these transformations is that without further modification, they are not successful with negative skewness or kurtosis.[8] Such conditions are not usually found in observations of clinical laboratory analytes, but they do occur occasionally. Moreover, Harris and DeMets did not mention the need for formal goodness-of-fit tests to judge agreement of the transformed data with Normal form. The choice of first-stage transform and the decision to proceed to the inverse hyperbolic sine was left to the user, guided by the values of g_1 and g_2 obtained. Although these statistics are very helpful, they do not in themselves provide a reliable goodness-of-fit test for the Normal distribution.

Reed and Wu (1974) tested these transformations against a series of six simulated χ^2 (chi-square) distributions with degrees of freedom 2, 4, 6, 8, 10, and 20. The lowest degrees of freedom correspond to distributions with markedly positive skewness and kurtosis. The chi-square form approaches the Normal as the degrees of freedom increase, so that a χ^2 distribution with 20 degrees of freedom is almost symmetric. Comparing the means and standard deviations of sample quantiles and Normal estimators (after transformation) at $p = 0.025$ and $p = 0.975$ over 25 independent samples of 100 observations from each of these chi-square distributions, Reed and Wu found the

---

[7] The hyperbolic sine function of a variable x is defined by $\sinh(x) = (e^x + e^{-x})/2$. The inverse function $y = \sinh^{-1}(x) = \log_e[x + (x^2 + 1)^{1/2}] = \int dx/(x^2 + 1)^{1/2}$. Explicit equations for estimating δ and λ were given in Harris and DeMets (1972b, Appendix).

[8] Negative skewness can be remedied by choosing a value of m greater than 2, so that $1 - m/2$ is negative. This leaves $m = 2$, the log transform, as a point of discontinuity, a mathematical problem avoided in the Box-Cox transform mentioned later.

Normal estimators to be more precise and slightly more accurate than the simple quantiles for almost symmetrical distributions, but less precise and slightly less accurate for skewed distributions.

Boyd and Lacher (1982) sought to correct the defects of the Harris-DeMets system of transformations while retaining the two-stage feature. They supported the $\log(x + C)$ transform for both positive and negative skewness, proposing that negatively skewed data be multiplied by -1 to yield a mirror image of a positively skewed distribution to which the $\log(x + C)$ transform could then be applied. For removal of residual negative kurtosis, they suggested the hyperbolic sine function rather than its inverse, incorporating a scaling constant into both forms. In addition, they proposed a new second-stage transform, a power function $|z|^K$ for $z \geq 0$ and $-|z|^K$ for $z < 0$ (z being the standardized transformed value after the first stage). For positive kurtosis, K would lie between 0 and 1; for negative kurtosis, K would exceed 1. After determining K iteratively (like C in the log transform), Boyd and Lacher suggested modifying K to $K' = (K + 1)/2$.

Applying this transform system to real data sets for 20 common biochemical analytes, including enzymes that typically show highly skewed distributions, Boyd and Lacher found it to be successful in converting all distributions to Normal form as judged by a number of goodness-of-fit tests, including the Kolmogorov-Smirnov, Cramer–von Mises and Anderson-Darling tests (see Linnet, 1988, for a recent review and discussion of these tests). In addition, simulating the same chi-square distributions as did Reed and Wu (except for the chi-square with two degrees of freedom, which is the exponential distribution), drawing 25 random samples of 120 observations from each, they found the nonparametric estimate and two-stage log–hyperbolic sine transform yielded biased estimates, on average, while the log–power combination gave unbiased estimates. Both transform procedures resulted in Normal estimators with smaller variances (mean square errors) than shown by the sample quantile for all the simulated chi-square distributions.

We mentioned earlier some results obtained by Shultz et al. (1985) applying the Harrell-Davis weighted quantile procedure to simulations of eight model distributions. These authors also tested the efficiency of Normal estimators of $\zeta_{0.025}$ and $\zeta_{0.975}$ based on Boyd and Lacher's log–power transform procedure compared to the sample quantiles $Q_{0.025}$ and $Q_{0.975}$, drawing 1000 randomly generated samples of 119 observations per sample from each distribution form. Four of the mathematical distributions were highly atypical of clinical chemistry data, including U-shaped, rectangular, and exponential forms; the other four models were either more or less symmetrical or positively skewed (for example, one of these was the χ^2 distribution with four degrees of freedom.

In three of these latter models, the ratio of the variance of estimation using the Normal estimator after log–power transformation to the variance of the sample quantile averaged 70 percent, much greater than the expected ratio of variances when a Normal estimator is compared to the sample quantile in a truly Normal distribution (41 percent for the extreme percentiles estimated here). Recent work by Linnet (1987, 1988), described later, helps to explain the reason for this discrepancy. In the remaining model, the log–power transform did much worse than the quantile. However, this model, although fairly symmetric, was extremely peaked and closely bound on both ends. On the other hand, the Harrell-Davis method worked well on all four models, showing a variance ratio of 75 percent compared to the sample quantile, slightly better than the 80 percent expected from the simulation studies of Sheather and Marron (1990) mentioned earlier.

2.5.2 Methods from the Statistical Literature

The papers of Harris and DeMets (1972b), Reed and Wu (1974), Boyd and Lacher (1982), and Shultz et al. (1985) were all concerned with the role of Normalizing transforms in the determination of 95 percent reference limits for analytes commonly measured in clinical laboratories. Indeed, they were all published in the same journal, *Clinical Chemistry*. To a large extent, they represented arguments between proponents of parametric or nonparametric methods for estimating population percentiles and their confidence limits. While this debate was going on, however, a series of papers in the statistical literature was discussing in far greater mathematical detail the properties and relative merits of various transforms in serving more general statistical purposes (e.g., satisfying the assumptions of the analysis of variance regarding the additivity of effects, the constant variance of residuals, and their Normal distribution).

The Box-Cox Transforms

Most widely used of these transforms is the power function proposed by Box and Cox (1964),[9]

$$z(\lambda) = (x^\lambda - 1)/\lambda, \quad \text{for } \lambda \neq 0,$$
$$= \log x, \quad \text{for } \lambda = 0,$$

$$(2.4)$$

effective for removing skewness, either positive ($\lambda > 0$) or negative ($\lambda < 0$). The form of Equations (2.4), in contrast to $z = x^\lambda$, avoids discontinuity as λ passes from positive through zero to negative values. However, once an estimate of λ has been obtained, the simpler form $z = x^\lambda$ may be used since a linear function of a Normally distributed variable will also be Normal.

Box and Cox obtained a likelihood function for estimating λ by assuming that the transformed variable would be Normally distributed. This led to the maximized log likelihood function,

$$L_{max}(\lambda) = (-n/2) \log \sigma^2(\lambda) + (\lambda - 1) \Sigma \log x_i \qquad (2.5)$$

where $\sigma^2(\lambda)$ is the estimated variance of $z(\lambda)$ for given λ. As various writers have pointed out [e.g., Cole (1988)], this function is very close to a quadratic curve for $-1 \leq \lambda \leq +1$, the

---

[9] Not to be confused with the function $|z|^\kappa$ proposed by Boyd and Lacher (1982) as a second-stage transform to remove residual kurtosis.

range of greatest interest. Therefore, the maximum likelihood estimate (mle) of λ may be obtained with sufficient accuracy by computing $L_{max}(\lambda)$ for each of three values of λ spanning this range. Fitting the quadratic $L_{max}(\lambda) = a + b\lambda + c\lambda^2$, the mle is given by $-b/2c$, the maximum of the curve. Computation is simplest when the three values $\lambda = -1, 0, +1$ are chosen, in which case $\hat{\lambda} = (M_- - M_+)/2(M_- - 2M_0 + M_+)$, where M_-, M_0, and M_+ denote the values of the right-hand side of Equation (2.5) when $\lambda = -1, 0$, and $+1$, respectively. A BASIC program to compute the mle of λ in this way is listed in the Appendix 2.1. Applications to the ALT data and a serum haptoglobin data set are discussed in Section 2.5.4.

The Log(x + C) Transform

As noted earlier, the log transform has often been found to greatly reduce the skewness and kurtosis of the original distribution, but not achieve the symmetry of the bell-shaped curve. Further improvement may be obtained by adding a constant C to the values before taking logs. If positive skewness remains after the log transform, C should be negative (but $|C| < x_{(1)}$, the smallest observation); if negative skewness remains, C should be positive. Box and Cox included the transform log ($x + C$) as a special case of the extended power function,

$$z(\lambda, C) = [(x + C)^\lambda - 1]/\lambda, \quad \text{for } \lambda \neq 0, \qquad (2.6)$$
$$= \log(x + C), \quad \text{for } \lambda = 0.$$

The second term on the right-hand side of Equation (2.5) then becomes $(\lambda - 1) \Sigma \log(x + C)$. It turns out, however, as pointed out by Griffiths (1980), that for the shifted log transform ($\lambda = 0$), $L_{max}(0, C)$ is not quadratic around the mle of C and may, in fact, be quite flat. Griffiths demonstrated that the function is much closer to quadratic when plotted not against C but against $\eta = -\log(x_{(1)} + C)$. Using this change of scale allows the mle of C to be computed in much the same way as λ in the simple power transform. A BASIC program for this purpose starting with the initial estimate $\hat{C} = 0$ is listed in Appendix 2.1.[10] The final value of $\hat{C}$ should be tested by computing the coefficients of skewness and kurtosis under the transform $\log(x + \hat{C})$ and plotting the transformed distribution on Normal probability paper. Results for the ALT data are included in Section 2.5.4.

Manly's Exponential Transform and John and Draper's Modulus Function

Manly (1976) suggested an alternative to the Box-Cox transform

$$z(\gamma) = [\exp(\gamma x) - 1]/\gamma, \qquad \gamma \neq 0,$$
$$= x, \gamma = 0. \tag{2.7}$$

on the grounds that, unlike the Box-Cox transform, the exponential form allows negative values of x. This would not seem to offer any advantage in laboratory medicine. The maximum likelihood estimating formula cannot be solved explicitly, but

---

[10] Royston (1992) has suggested that since the goal of the transform $\log(x + C)$ is to produce a symmetric distribution, the ratio

$$\frac{\log(x_{(n)} + C) - \log(x_{\text{med}} + C)}{\log(x_{\text{med}} + C) - \log(x_{(1)} + C)}$$

where $x_{(1)}$, x_{med} and $x_{(n)}$ are, respectively, the smallest, median and largest observations, should equal unity. This leads to an inital estimate of

$$\hat{C} = \frac{x_{(1)}x_{(n)} - x_{\text{med}}^2}{x_{(1)} + x_{(n)} - 2x_{\text{med}}}$$

This may prove a better starting point than $\hat{C} = 0$ when the skewness remaining after the simple log transform is relatively high, but is subject to the vagaries of extreme observations. One possibility is to compute this ratio for paired values $x_{(1)},x_{(n)}$; $x_{(2)},x_{(n-1)}$; $x_{(3)},x_{(n-2)}$, and average the results, assuming that none of these pairs produces a negative estimate of C such that $|\hat{C}|$ exceeds $x_{(1)}$.

Manly helps to overcome this difficulty through the inverse transformation

$$x = \log_e(1 + \gamma z)/\gamma, \quad \gamma \neq 0,$$
$$= z, \quad \gamma = 0. \tag{2.8}$$

Assuming that the exponential transform produces a Normal distribution with mean zero and standard deviation unity, he applies this inverse transform to standard Normal deviates and calculates the mean, standard deviation, and coefficients of skewness and kurtosis of the original variate x. These parameters are tabulated for each of a series of γ values from 0 to 0.5 at intervals of 0.05. Through this table (Manly, 1976 Table 1), the user may relate estimates of these parameters from the data to the appropriate value of γ. An example is given.

The Box-Cox and Manly transform functions are intended particularly to remove the effects of skewness in the original data. As we discussed earlier, there may still be residual kurtosis. We referred then to the proposal by Boyd and Lacher (1982) that this problem might be resolved through the second-stage transform $|z|^K$ for $z \geq 0$ and $-|z|^K$ for $z < 0$, where z is the standardized transformed value after the first stage. In the statistical literature, John and Draper (1980) proposed the same function, but defined the power K as equal to $\hat{\lambda}$ derived from the Box-Cox transform. Thus, if the Box-Cox transform is used to remove skewness and at least some if not all kurtosis, the function proposed by John and Draper (which they called the *modulus* function) may achieve this last Normalizing task without the need to estimate a new parameter. However, using the Box-Cox estimate of $\hat{\lambda} < 1$, the modulus function would work for positive but not negative kurtosis. The Boyd-Lacher proposal (including the hyperbolic sine transform) would deal with either type.

The Expert Panel on Theory of Reference Values of the International Federation of Clinical Chemistry (1987) has considered all the transformation functions described above. The panel favors the concept of a two-stage transformation, recommending for this purpose Manly's exponential transform to remove positive or negative skewness, followed, if necessary by the modulus function of John and Draper to eliminate any residual (positive) kurtosis. The Anderson-Darling goodness-of-fit test is recommended to test final agreement with a Normal distribution. Programs to estimate the transforming parameters and to carry out various goodness-of-fit tests have been included in the document REFVAL, prepared in 1983 by Solberg, the panel's last chairman.

We are of the opinion that a Box-Cox power function [including $\log(x + C)$] as a first-stage transform followed, if necessary, by the modulus function makes a more natural pair, assuming positive kurtosis. On the other hand, the Boyd-Lacher second-stage power transform would deal with any residual significant negative kurtosis at the cost of estimating another parameter.

2.5.3 More Recent Analyses of Transformation Procedures

We have not considered confidence interval estimates of transformation parameters, but only point estimates. Our reasons are not only to avoid additional mathematical complexities, but also because in practical calculations of reference limits, information about the precision of point estimates of these parameters seems to us irrelevant. For example, the square root transform would be used whenever $\hat{\lambda}$ lies in the range 0.45–0.55. Similarly, the log transform would be applied whenever $\hat{\lambda}$ lies within ± 0.1.

However, Linnet (1987, 1988) has shown that the statistical variability of estimates of transformation parameters has a significant effect on the actual (as opposed to theoretical) efficiency of parametric estimation of reference limits. Rather than starting with known non-Normal distributions as have previous authors in the clinical literature, Linnet followed Manly's approach by generating random samples from a theoretical Normal distribution and then subjecting the numbers in each sample to a two-stage inverse transformation process. Starting with the John-

Draper modulus function followed by Box and Cox's or Manly's transformation functions, Linnet selected transformation parameters to achieve a moderately skewed distribution typical of many biochemical analytes. The author then proceeded to apply these transformations in the usual order as if the original transformation parameters were unknown, iterating as necessary to find those values of the (two-stage) transformation parameters that reduced the coefficients of skewness and kurtosis to zero in each random sample. A total of 1000 independent random Normal samples were drawn, each containing 119 numbers.

Linnet computed two Normal estimators of $\zeta_{0.975}$ for each random sample, one from the original random Normal values, the second from the values obtained after applying the inverse-forward transformation for that sample. He found that the standard deviation of the second set of estimators over all samples was 25 percent greater than the standard deviation of estimators from the original samples. The sampling variation of estimated transformation parameters had increased the sampling variance of Normal estimators of $\zeta_{0.975}$ by a factor of $(1.25)^2$, or 1.56. From this we infer that the relative efficiency of the quantile estimator $Q_{0.975}$ compared to the Normal estimator increases from 41 percent in the case of a Normal distribution to a probable value of 100(1.56/2.44), or 64 percent, in typically skewed distributions to which the recommended two-stage transformation process has been applied. This latter figure agrees reasonably well with the average of 70 percent efficiency of sample quantiles mentioned above as found by Shultz et al. (1985) in similar distributions where the log–power transformation of Boyd and Lacher was applied.

Further, Linnet (1988) showed that the sampling variation in estimates of transformation parameters causes the usual goodness-of-fit tests of the transformed distributions (Anderson-Darling, Cramer–von Mises, or Kolmogorov-Smirnov tests) to be too conservative in their assessments. That is, they fail to reject the hypothesis of Normal form, using the 0.05 level of significance, as often as they should, so that the transformation process appears to achieve Normality more frequently than it really does. The author provides correction factors (depending on sample size) for these tests.

When the Harrell-Davis estimator is used instead of the simple quantile, the efficiency of estimation in typically skewed distributions may be expected to rise to about 77 percent (64 × 1.2), compared to the Normal estimator after transformation, assuming the transformation process succeeds in producing a Normal distribution. In view of the foregoing results, and the ease of computerized bootstrap estimation, this nonparametric approach would seem to be the method of choice for estimating reference limits and their confidence intervals. Nevertheless, as the following examples prove, the asymmetric distributions of some (perhaps many) analytes can be easily converted to essentially Normal form through the Box-Cox transforms. In such cases, and particularly when estimates of various percentiles of the population are desired, the advantages of the Normal estimator are clear. We meet the same issue of nonparametric versus parametric estimation in computing time-dependent reference ranges, discussed in Chapter 5.

2.5.4 Examples

Two data sets are listed in Appendix 2.1: (1) alanine aminotransferase (ALT), referred to earlier in this chapter, and (2) serum haptoglobin, reported by Reed et al. (1971). Table 2.2 lists the statistics of these data, the sample quantiles $Q_{0.025}$ and $Q_{0.975}$, the mean quantiles using the bootstrapped Harrell-Davis procedure, and 90 percent confidence intervals for $\zeta_{0.025}$ and $\zeta_{0.975}$ under each method of estimation.

The reference limits agree closely under both methods, except for the lower limit in haptoglobin. In this case, the sample quantile $Q_{0.025}$ is low because of two occurrences of 21 mg/100 mL at the low end of the data, reflecting the sensitivity of extreme quantiles when the total sample size is not too large. If we disregard the open-endedness of the haptoglobin intervals based on the sample quantiles, the bootstrap confidence inter-

Table 2.2 Analysis of ALT and Haptoglobin Data

A. Statistics of the observed data

Analyte	n	Mean	SD	g_1	g_2
ALT (U/L)	240	22.5	11.9	1.34	1.75
Serum haptoglobin (mg/100 ml)	100	95.3	42.7	0.64	0.31

B. Quantiles and nonparametric 90 percent confidence intervals

Analyte	$Q_{0.025}$	Conf. interval	$Q_{0.975}$	Conf. interval
ALT				
Sample quantile	8	6–9	54	49–65
Bootstrap	7.7 (mean)	6.3–9.1	53.8 (mean)	48.4–58.1
Serum haptoglobin				
Sample quantile	21	<14–35[a]	194	176–>225[a]
Bootstrap	26.0	14.6–37.3	191.2	168–214

[a] These intervals were obtained using the approximate method. Under this method, the smallest value of n allowing specific calculation of the lower 90 percent confidence limit for $\zeta_{0.025}$ or the upper 90 percent confidence limit for $\zeta_{0.975}$ is 143.

vals were only slightly if at all narrower, except at the upper limit of the reference range for ALT. A more important advantage than narrower confidence intervals is the fact that bootstrapped intervals can be determined even for the relatively small sample sizes that may be necessary for special populations such as neonates or infants.

Turning to parametric (Normal) estimators, and using the method described earlier (and the BASIC program listed in Appendix 2.1), the mle of the Box-Cox power parameter λ for the ALT data was −0.052, indicating the log transform, and for haptoglobin, 0.53, indicating the square root transform. The small amounts of skewness and kurtosis remaining in the distribution of log (ALT) were almost completely removed by the transform log (ALT − 1.6); the mle $\hat{C}$ = −1.6 was obtained using the second BASIC program listed in the appendix. Table 2.3 presents the statistics of the data on these transformed scales, the Normal estimators of $\zeta_{0.025}$ and $\zeta_{0.975}$ and the corresponding 90 percent confidence intervals. On the transformed scale, the estimators are $\bar{x} \pm 1.96s$, and the confidence intervals are $\hat{\zeta}_{0.025}$ or $\hat{\zeta}_{0.975} \pm (1.645)(2.92/n)^{1/2}SD$.

Table 2.3 Analysis of $\log_e$ (ALT), $\log_e$ (ALT − 1.6), and (Haptoglobin)$^{1/2}$

A. Statistics of the transformed data

Analyte	Mean	SD	g_1	g_2	Shapiro-Wilk test[a] P-value
$\log_e$ (ALT)	2.99	0.496	0.11	−0.14	0.15
$\log_e$ (ALT − 1.6)	2.89	0.545	−0.044	0.019	0.25
sqrt (haptoglobin)	9.51	2.23	−0.03	0.05	0.68

B. Normal estimators and 90 percent confidence intervals after back-transformation

Analyte	$\zeta_{0.025}$	Conf. interval	$\zeta_{0.975}$	Conf. interval
ALT[b]	7.8	7.2–8.4	54.1	49.2–59.6
Haptoglobin	26.4	20.4–33.3	192.3	175.4–210.1

[a] The Shapiro-Wilk test for agreement with a Normal distribution is part of the SAS programming system (PROC UNIVARIATE) that was used to obtain these statistics. It is well known as a powerful test for Normality.

[b] The estimate of $\zeta_{0.025}$, for example, is obtained by calculating $\bar{y} - 1.96s = Q'$, say, where $\bar{y}$ and s are the mean and standard deviation of log (ALT − 1.6), then computing $e^{Q'} + 1.6$. Similarly, upper and lower 90 percent confidence limits would be computed as $Q' \pm 1.645 (2.92/n)^{1/2}s$, then exponentiating these limits and adding 1.6.

Figure 2.3 shows a graph of the data (ALT − 1.6) on log-Normal paper. The approximate linearity indicates good fit of a logNormal distribution function. For both analytes, the Normal estimates of the reference limits agree well with the nonparametric bootstrap estimates. The greater precision of the para-

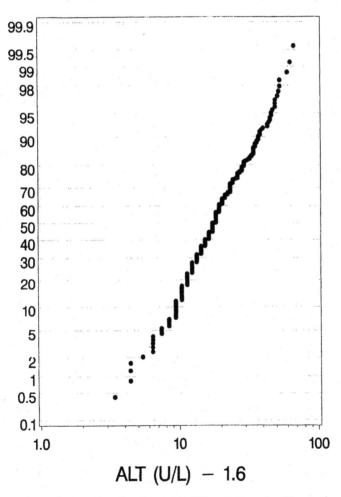

Fig. 2.3 Cumulative distribution of (ALT − 1.6) on logNormal probability paper.

metric analysis shows in the confidence intervals, with one exception: the width of the interval for $\xi_{0.975}$ in ALT is about the same under the Normally distributed transform as when the bootstrap method is used. Otherwise, the widths of 90 percent confidence intervals using the transforms are much narrower, averaging only about 60 percent of the widths of intervals under the bootstrap procedure.

Interestingly, for each analyte, the width of the Normal-based 90 percent confidence interval for $\zeta_{0.975}$ is 21–22 percent of the 95 percent reference range. It turns out that the numbers of reference subjects sampled (240 for ALT, 100 for haptoglobin) are just slightly below the sample sizes required to achieve a relative width of 20 percent in each case. In the next chapter, we pursue the topic of recommended sample sizes for reference range estimation.

APPENDIX 2.1   BASIC PROGRAM FOR mle OF BOX-COX POWER PARAMETER λ

```
10 REM PROGR. FOR MLE BOX-COX POWER

20 OPEN "LPT1:" FOR OUTPUT AS #1

30 DIM X(500),M(3)

40 N=sample size, supplied by user

50 FOR Q=1 TO 3

60 L=Q-2

70 R=0

80 S=0

90 T=0

100 V=0

110 FOR I=1 TO N
```

```
120 READ X(I)

130 Y=LOG (X(I))

140 S=S+Y

150 IF L=0 GOTO 200

160 W=((X(I)^L)-1)/L

170 T=T+W

180 V=V+W*W

190 GOTO 210

200 R=R+Y*Y

210 NEXT I

220 RESTORE

230 IF L=0 GOTO 300

240 V=V-(T*T)/N

250 V=V/N

260 A=(-N/2)*LOG(V)

270 B=(L-1)*S

280 M(Q)=A+B

290 GO TO 340

300 R=R-(S*S)/N

310 R=R/N

320 A=(-N/2)*LOG(R)

330 M(Q)=A-S

340 PRINT #1, "POWER=",L

350 PRINT #1, "M(L)=",M(Q)
```

```
360 PRINT #1,

370 NEXT Q

380 L1=M(1)-M(3)

390 L2=M(1)-2*M(2)+M(3)

400 L=L1/(2*L2)

410 PRINT #1, "MLE OF POWER=",L

500 DATA
```

APPENDIX 2.2 BASIC PROGRAM FOR mle OF *C* IN TRANSFORM log(*x* + *C*)

```
10 REM PROGR. FOR MLE OF C IN LOG (X + C)

20 OPEN "LPT1:" FOR OUTPUT AS #1

30 DIM X(300),M(3)

40 N=sample size, supplied by user

50 K=1 (or 2, see note below)

60 C=0

70 U1= (x(1), the smallest observation, supplied by user)

80 E=-LOG (U1 + C)

90 FOR Q=1 TO 3

100 L=K*(Q-2) + E

110 C=EXP (-L) - U1

120 S=0

130 T=0

140 FOR I=1 TO N
```

```
150 READ X(I)

160 Y=LOG (X(I) + C)

170 S=S + Y

180 T=T + Y*Y

190 NEXT I

200 RESTORE

210 V=T - (S*S)/N

220 V=V/N230 A=(-N/2)*LOG (V)

240 M(Q)=A - S

250 PRINT #1, "E(L)=",L

260 PRINT #1, "M(E)=",M(Q)

270 PRINT #1,

280 NEXT Q

290 F1=M(1) - M(3)

300 F2=M(1) - 2*M(2) + M(3)

310 F=F1/(2*F2)

320 F=K*F + E

330 PRINT #1, "MLE OF E=",F

340 C1=EXP (-F) - U1

350 PRINT #1, "MLE OF C=", C1

500 DATA
```

APPENDIX 2.3 DATA SETS

A2.3.1 Frequency Distribution of Alanine Aminotransferase (ALT) in 240 Medical Students

Value (U/L)	Frequency	Value	Frequency
5	1	31	5
6	3	32	1
7	1	33	1
8	5	34	2
9	3	35	2
10	4	36	6
11	11	37	3
12	13	38	2
13	13	39	3
14	13	40	3
15	10	41	1
16	11	42	1
17	9	45	2
18	10	46	1
19	13	47	2
20	15	48	2
21	11	49	1
22	8	51	3
23	5	53	1
24	3	54	1
25	11	55	2
26	5	62	1
27	1	65	1
28	6	69	1
29	2		
30	5		

Source: Department of Pathology, University of Virginia Health Sciences Center, Charlottesville, Virginia.

A2.3.2 Frequency Distribution of Serum Haptoglobin (mg/100 ml, as hemoglobin-binding capacity)

14	59	82	100	128
21	62	84	100	129
21	65	85	101	135
30	66	86	101	136
32	67	87	101	141
35	67	87	103	142
36	69	88	105	147
36	71	88	106	147
40	72	89	108	150
44	76	90	108	161
47	76	90	108	162
48	77	93	109	170
48	77	94	113	174
48	77	94	114	174
50	77	95	114	176
51	78	96	114	179
52	79	96	116	181
54	79	97	116	191
58	80	98	119	199
59	81	98	126	225

Source: Reed et al. (1971), Table 1.

3

SAMPLE SIZES AND SUBGROUPS

3.1 HOW MANY SUBJECTS?

3.1.1 Introduction

Official documents on the subject of reference ranges (e.g., the reports of the IFCC Expert Panel on Reference Values) devote much more attention to criteria for selection and treatment of reference subjects than they do to the recommended number of subjects. This is not unreasonable because a relatively small but demographically homogeneous group of subjects provides a more useful reference range, if applied to patients having the same characteristics, than does a large collection of persons with highly varied demographic characteristics. Moreover, unless certain rules of pre-analytical behavior and treatment of subjects are followed, the resulting measurements may be more misleading than helpful.

Nevertheless, given the large role played by sample size in determining the precision with which reference limits are estimated, we must give this topic more than usual consideration. Indeed, within the context of reference ranges, there are few papers in the literature discussing in detail the appropriate number of subjects for estimating cross-sectional reference limits. As noted in Chapter 1, numbers of subjects in past studies have varied widely, from less than 100 in earlier days to several thousand in later years when blood sampling was undertaken as part of health screening programs. A recent publication (Ueland et al., 1993) presents a frequency distribution reproduced in Figure 3.1 of total plasma homocysteine values in 3000 men, aged 40–42 years!

In the preceding chapter we considered the relative efficiency of nonparametric estimates of reference limits compared to the Normal estimator when the distribution of values in the sampled population conformed to the Normal curve. For example, if no transformation of scale is required, the simple quantile estimates of the percentiles $\zeta_{0.025}$ or $\zeta_{0.975}$ are only 41 percent as efficient as the Normal estimators $\bar{x} \pm 1.96s$. As noted earlier, Linnet (1987) demonstrated that the efficiency of the nonpara-

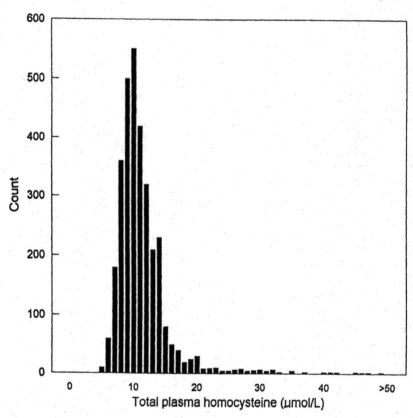

Fig. 3.1 Distribution of plasma homocysteine values in 3000 men, aged 40–42. (From Ueland et al., 1993, with permission.)

metric estimator increases when a transformation is needed to obtain a Normal distribution of values. When the bootstrap (weighted percentile) method of Harrell and Davis is used, the efficiency of nonparametric estimation increases again. In any case, however, efficiency is only a relative index, not sufficient by itself to determine the minimum number of subjects required for a confidence interval of specified width. For this, we need an additional criterion.

For example, Reed et al. (1971), who favored the nonparametric quantile estimator because of the complexity of finding the best transforming function to produce a Normal distribution, and the uncertainty of success, suggested a minimum of 120 subjects. As noted in Chapter 2, this is the smallest number for which one may obtain exact nonparametric 90 percent confidence intervals (based on order statistics) for the true percentiles being estimated. Using the Normal approximation formulas given in Section (2.2.2), a minimum of 143 subjects is required.

Miller et al. (1984) developed an empirical criterion for the minimum number of subjects based on computerized sampling from a highly skewed distribution. Working with creatine kinase values in 379 women, these authors tried six different mathematical models in an attempt to fit the observed distribution. They were unsuccessful in every case, using the Kolmogorov-Smirnov goodness-of-fit test. They did not look specifically for a Normalizing transformation function of the kind discussed in Chapter 2, although one of the mathematical models they considered was the logNormal. Turning to nonparametric estimation, the authors carried out what amounted to a kind of bootstrap sampling of the observed distribution, although they did not use this term.

Drawing sets of 500 random samples, with replacement, of 100, 200, 400, and 800 observations per sample, they computed the mean and standard deviation of the sample quantile $Q_{0.975}$ for each set of 500 resamples. (In bootstrap sampling, the number of values in each resample typically equals n, the size of the original sample.) The value of $Q_{0.975}$ in the original sample of 379 observations was 240 U/L. The mean values of $Q_{0.975}$ in 100, 200, 400, and 800 observations per resample were 259, 260, 248, and 242 U/L, respectively, and the corresponding standard deviations were 64, 57, 43, and 35 U/L. The declining standard deviations, with some tapering off after 400 observations, led Miller et al. to conclude that samples of less than 200 subjects are inadequate to define 95 percent reference limits for highly skewed distributions, using the quantile estimator, but that a sample size of 400 would be acceptable. Moreover, outlying observations in samples of size 100 or 200 that might have been rejected as contaminants from another distribution were found in the larger samples to fit comfortably within the tail of a single highly skewed but homogeneous distribution.

It is unfortunate that, except for the log function, Miller et al. did not try any of the transform functions suggested by earlier writers to see whether they might have produced at least approximately Normal forms. Although the Normal estimator will still be somewhat biased after back-transforming to original units (since exact agreement with the Normal form is not possible with real data), its precision is so much greater than the simple quantile estimator that it could be associated with a confidence interval lying *within* the nonparametric interval derived from the same sample of observations. In the ALT example in Chapter 2, this result held in the confidence intervals for $\zeta_{0.025}$ and almost, but not quite, in the confidence intervals for $\zeta_{0.975}$ (compare Tables 2.2b and 2.3b).

The work of Miller et al. indicated that when sample quantiles are used, sample sizes of at least several hundred subjects are required to estimate the 95 percent reference limits of highly skewed distributions with acceptable precision. However, these results do not provide a general criterion for determining the minimum sample sizes needed to obtain acceptably accurate estimates (parametric or nonparametric) of the desired reference limits in either Normal or skewed distributions. For progress in this direction, we turn to more recent work by Linnet (1987).

3.1.2 A General Criterion for Sample Size

Linnet cited the rule that analytical variation should be small compared to biological variation. By analogy, he argued that the sample size should be large enough to make the width of the 90 percent confidence interval for a reference limit small compared to the width of the 95 percent reference range. He suggested possible ratios of 0.1, 0.2, or 0.3 for these two widths and computed as base figures, the numbers of subjects required to achieve these values for a Normal distribution using the Normal estimator of $\zeta_{0.975}$. To illustrate this calculation for the ratio $R = 0.2$, we note that:

1. Since the 95 percent reference range is $\bar{x} \pm 1.96s$, its width equals $3.92s$;

2. The Normal estimator of $\zeta_{0.975}$ is $\bar{x} + 1.96s$. Its large-sample variance is estimated by $(s^2/n)[1 + (1.96)^2/2] = 2.92s^2/n$, so that the width of the 90 percent confidence interval for $\zeta_{0.975}$ is $2(1.645)(s/n^{1/2})(1.709)$, or $5.623 \, s/n^{1/2}$;

3. Then, R, the ratio of these widths, equals $1.434/n^{1/2}$;

4. For $R = 0.2$, $n = 51.4$, or 52.

We have already seen that when the population distribution is Normal, the quantile estimator $Q_{0.975}$ would require 2.44 times 51.4, or $n = 126$ subjects to attain the same precision of estimation. Since the efficiency of the Harrell-Davis bootstrap estimator is about 20 percent greater than that of the quantile, or about 51 percent of the Normal estimator, assuming a Normal distribution, the corresponding sample size using the bootstrap estimator is $n = 101$. If R were set equal to 0.1 instead of 0.2, the minimal sample sizes would all be much higher: 206 for the Normal estimator, 502 for the sample quantile, and 404 for the bootstrap estimator.

The problem becomes more complicated when the sampled population is not Normal but skewed. Linnet's basic approach may still be applied, however; that is, after transforming the measurements to a Normal scale, determine the sample size using the Normal estimator for a specified value of R and then adjust this sample size for nonparametric estimation by dividing by the efficiency of the nonparametric estimator relative to the Normal estimator.

To start with, consider a skewed distribution that can be transformed to Normal form (at least to a close approximation) through the square root transformation $y = x^{1/2}$, as in the hapto-globin example given in Chapter 2. We would use the Normal estimators to obtain upper and lower reference limits, and back-transform to the original (x) scale by squaring these limits. Then, the width of the 95 percent reference range, say $W_{r.r.}$, will be

$$W_{r.r.} = (\bar{y} + 1.96s_y)^2 - (\bar{y} - 1.96s_y)^2$$
$$= 4\bar{y}s_y(1.96), \tag{3.1}$$

where $\bar{y}$ is the mean and s_y the standard deviation of the square roots.

Similarly, the width of the 90 percent confidence interval for $\zeta_{0.975}$ will be the difference between the square of the upper limit of the confidence interval (computed from the Normal esti-mator) minus the square of the lower limit. Carrying through the algebra,[1] the width of the confidence interval on the original scale, say $W_{c.i.}$ may be written as

$$W_{c.i.} = 4ys_y\, 2.811(1 + 1.96C_y)/n^{1/2}, \tag{3.2}$$

where C_y is the coefficient of variation (standard deviation di-vided by the mean) of the distribution of the square roots. Di-viding $W_{c.i.}$ by $W_{r.r.}$, we obtain $R = (1/n^{1/2})(1.434 + 2.811C_y)$. Setting $R = 0.2$, say, and inserting a value of C_y, we can solve for the required sample size n. For example, if $C_y = 0.2$ (20 percent), and we set $R = 0.2$, then the minimal number of

---

[1] On the original scale, the widths of the reference range and the confidence interval around the upper percentile are of the form $F = (a + b)^{1/m} - (a - b)^{1/m}$, where m is the parameter in the transform $y = x^m$. For $m = \frac{1}{2}$, $F = 4ab$; for $m = \frac{1}{3}$ and $\frac{1}{4}$, and large sample sizes $(n \geq 100)$, F is closely approximated by $6a^2b$ and $8a^3b$, respectively, eliminating the need for trial-and-error solutions for n at these values of m.

subjects required is 100. But if C_y = 0.6, the required number becomes 244. In the haptoglobin data of Chapter 2, C_y = 0.23, so the number of subjects actually sampled in this case (100) was close to the number 109 calculated by setting R equal to 0.2. As we saw, the relative width (R) of the 90 percent confidence interval for $\zeta_{0.975}$ in the distribution of serum haptoglobin was 21 percent.

Figure 3.2 plots the required sample sizes to obtain R = 0.2 for a range of values of C_y when the exponent m in the normalizing power transform $y = x^m$ is equal to $\frac{1}{2}$, $\frac{1}{3}$, or $\frac{1}{4}$, that

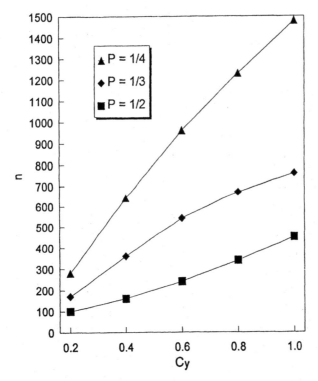

Fig. 3.2 Sample size needed to estimate 97.5 percent reference limit with confidence interval 20 percent as wide as 95 percent reference range, using square root, cube root, or fourth root transformation; C_y = CV on transformed scale.

is, for distributions of increasing skewness. A BASIC program to calculate these sample sizes for any value of R is listed in Appendix 3.1.

The value $m = 0$ corresponds to the log transform $y = \log_e(x)$. A logNormal distribution for a biochemical analyte typically shows a large coefficient of variation on the original measurement scale. In such cases, one may expect that large sample sizes would be needed to achieve a 90 percent confidence interval for $\zeta_{0.975}$ no wider than 20 percent ($R = 0.2$) of the width of the 95 percent reference range. Figure 3.3 bears this out for

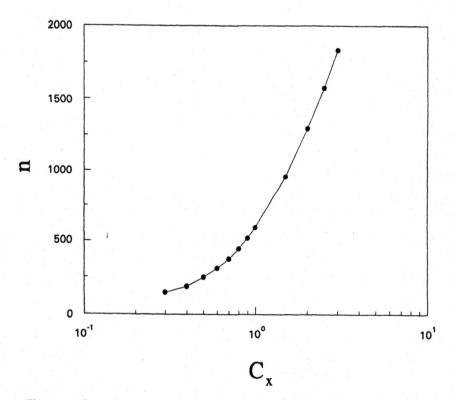

Fig. 3.3 Sample size needed to estimate 97.5 percent reference limit with confidence interval 20 percent as wide as 95 percent reference range, using log transform; C_x = CV on original scale.

values of C_x greater than 1. Note that for the log transform, the coefficient of variation on the original, not the transformed, scale is used to compute required sample sizes (see Appendix 3.1 for mathematical details).

In the ALT example, the sample size of 240 subjects was somewhat less than that recommended (266) by the graph in Figure 3.3 at the observed value of C_x (0.53). As expected, the width of the 90 percent parametric confidence interval for $\zeta_{0.975}$ in this example was slightly more than 20 percent of the width of the 95 percent reference range.

As noted in Section 2.5.3, Linnet concluded that when the transforming parameter needs to be estimated, the confidence interval for $\zeta_{0.975}$ using the Normal estimator should be widened by about 25 percent to account for sampling variation in the estimate of this parameter. This implies that in such cases the sample sizes shown in Figures 3.2 and 3.3 for Normal estimators should be increased by a factor of $(1.25)^2$, or 1.56. The sample sizes for nonparametric estimation would remain unchanged, so that, as we noted in Chapter 2, the efficiency of the simple quantile estimator would rise to 64 percent, and that of the Harrell-Davis bootstrap estimator to 77 percent. In other words, the comparable sample size for the quantile estimator would then be 1.56 times (1/0.64) as large as that for the Normal estimator, while the sample size for the bootstrap estimator would be 1.30 times as large (1/0.77).

In practice, the best transforming parameter might be readily apparent despite potential sampling variation in the estimates. This was the case in both the ALT and haptoglobin examples, where we found that the sample sizes employed performed exactly as expected from Figures 3.2 and 3.3; that is, slightly less than the sizes recommended by these graphs, they produced 90 percent parametric confidence intervals for $\zeta_{0.975}$ slightly wider than 20 percent of the corresponding reference ranges. We suggest, therefore, that in many real applications of transforming to Normal form and then back-transforming, the sample sizes indicated in these graphs will satisfy the specification of $R = 0.2$ without a 56 percent inflation factor.

In such cases, the theoretical efficiency of the Normal estimator would still hold.

3.1.3 Practical Implications

For the skewed distributions commonly found in biochemical analytes these recommended sample sizes depend on information that is not available until a considerable number of observations have already been obtained. Only then can the coefficient of variation on the original or transformed scale be estimated. However, measurements on large numbers of reference subjects are usually not collected all at once but over a period of time. It seems reasonable to suggest that after 150–200 subjects have been measured, the distribution of their results be examined and an estimate of the transformation parameter required to achieve a Normal distribution be obtained, for example, through the use of Equation (2.5). Then, the results given above may be applied to estimate the final number of subjects needed to reach the desired value of the ratio R.

3.2 INDIVIDUALIZING THE REFERENCE RANGE

As we noted in Chapter 1, the cross-sectional reference range has many conceptual defects, yet is so deeply ingrained in laboratory and clinical practice that it will probably remain a permanent fixture. A basic problem is that the biological variance reflected in the width of the reference range arises chiefly from variation in the biochemistries of individuals with diverse age, race, and gender characteristics. On the other hand, as Figure 3.1 shows, considerable variation may remain even when the sampled population is narrowly restricted on all these factors.

It is difficult, therefore, to escape the problem that cross-sectional reference ranges are obtained from a collective but applied to individuals. One alternative is the subject-specific reference range based on a series of measurements of the analyte in a given individual. In healthy individuals, these might be at annual or 6-month intervals, long enough to maintain statistical independence between successive results, yet allowing a number of observations within a time period short enough to avoid the interference of aging effects. Some theory of Bayesian predictive ranges based on simple, short time series models, developed in the decade from the mid-1970s to the mid-1980s, was summarized by Albert and Harris (1987, chap. 8). Without doubt, more widespread distribution of portable personalized medical records will accelerate the use of subject-specific predictive ranges in healthy individuals.

Application of time series methods in patients generally involves much more frequent sampling, as in monitoring tumor biomarkers following initial treatment (Winkel et al., 1982) or serum creatinine after renal transplant (Smith and West, 1983). Schlain et al. (1992, 1993) advanced this work in both theory and application through the study of autoregressive and random walk models applied to unequally spaced, correlated observations of biomarkers in women treated for breast cancer. This development is described in Chapter 7.

Other ways of "individualizing" cross-sectional reference ranges without abandoning the population base make use of the entire distribution of reference results, not merely the 95 percent limits. With modern methods of information transmission and storage, every clinical laboratory should be allowed easy access to these distributions regardless of where they have been obtained. As mentioned in Chapter 1, various authors have proposed that laboratories report not only the measured value of an analyte in a patient sample, but also the percentile of the reference distribution which that value represents. In this way, the atypicality of a result close to but not beyond the upper reference limit could be emphasized.

As an alternative to storing and searching the entire reference distribution for each analyte, a clinical laboratory might retain just the mean ($\bar{x}$) and standard deviation (s) of this distribution. Then, along with each result, its "SD unit" $z = (x - \bar{x})/s$ could be reported. This system was initially proposed by Gullick and Schauble (1972). A z value close to ± 2 would presumably sound an alarm when the clinician reviewed the report. The advantage of the SD unit lies in its independence of measurement units and the general familiarity of clinicians with ±2 as a statistical marker.

Although in theory, the SD unit would seem to assume a Normal distribution of reference values, in fact, for moderately skewed as well as symmetrical distributions, the mean ±2 standard deviations includes close to 95 percent of the observations. The SD unit could also be extended to multivariate distributions of analytes (Albert and Harris, 1987, pp. 65–67), but here the assumption of a multivariate Normal distribution is stronger. Moreover, in addition to the mean and standard deviation of each analyte, the covariances of all pairs of analytes would be needed.

Albert (1981) suggested extending the SD unit to an atypicality index defined as the probability (or rather, 1 minus the probability) that the observed result or profile of results is representative of the reference population (Albert and Harris, 1987, pp. 67–69). This index lies between 0 and 1, a value close to 1 indicating that the result is unlikely to have come from the reference population.

Finally, the likelihood ratio (Albert, 1982; Albert and Harris, 1987, pp. 82–96) compares the conditional probability of the observed result given that the patient belongs to one population (e.g., healthy) with the probability of the result given that the patient comes from another population (e.g., diseased). Of course, this requires knowledge of the distribution of reference values in both populations. Albert has developed a general exponential model for the likelihood ratio similar to the logistic model in discriminant analysis. In the univariate case, the coefficients of this model are expressible in terms of the sensitivity and specificity of the diagnostic test. The model easily generalizes to allow estimation of the likelihood ratio for a multivariate vector of test results.

All these various proposals (except for subject-specific ranges) focus on representing the status of a current patient relative to one (or two) reference population(s). As mentioned earlier, they require that each clinical laboratory either store reference distributions (or their basic statistics) in its own files or maintain ready access to this information, perhaps through some national or regional repository. This should become a reality for any laboratory equipped with a modem and multimegabyte disk storage. At this point, however, we turn to consider a less far-reaching alternative, namely, development of reference ranges for specified age, gender, or race subgroups of the general healthy population. Specifically, we discuss criteria for answering the question: How many subgroups?

3.3 HOW MANY SUBGROUPS?

Separate reference ranges for different demographic subgroups already exist, for example, by gender, with respect to calcium, creatine, and uric acid in serum, and hemoglobin and hematocrit; by age group and gender for cholesterol in various forms and triglycerides. Wong et al. (1983) have found substantial racial and gender differences in creatine kinase, and Sinton et al. (1986) have presented evidence favoring a separate reference range for alkaline phosphatase in premenopausal women. As cited in Chapter 1, studies during the 1970s revealed statistically significant (but not always consistent) differences by gender and/or age in many analytes. More recently, Siest and colleagues (1985) have published a comprehensive work on biological variations in reference values.

However, with exceptions as noted above, separate reference ranges for use in general clinical practice have not been advocated despite statistically significant differences reported in the literature. Two reasons may be suggested: First, separate reference ranges for the same analyte are expensive to obtain, requiring multiple sets of reference subjects, and to maintain in laboratory reports; second, small differences of no clinical importance between the mean values of subgroups will inevitably become statistically significant if the sample sizes are large enough. Adding to these arguments is the finding that separate reference ranges are not much narrower than the combined range unless the difference between mean values is far greater than the minimal difference necessary to achieve statistical significance. We demonstrated this in Chapter 1 with respect to the decrease of serum albumin with age in men.

A nonparametric proof of this result for two subgroups was given recently by Harris and Boyd (1990), leading to the formula,

$$z = (2n)^{1/2}[(1 - h)^{-2} - 1]^{1/2}, \tag{3.3}$$

where h is the proportional reduction in standard deviation due to partitioning a combined population into two subgroups, n is the assumed equal size of each subgroup, and z is the smallest value of the standard Normal deviate used to compare two mean values that is required to achieve the reduction h in standard deviation.[2] Table 3.1 lists the z values from Equation (3.3) required to obtain 10 percent and 20 percent reductions in standard deviations.

Clearly, for the kinds of sample sizes suggested in Figures 3.2 and 3.3, very large differences between subgroup means are required to achieve even relatively small reductions in standard deviation through partitioning into separate reference ranges. Such differences would almost certainly arise from clinically important distinctions in the physiology of the analyte.

In our earlier discussion about the recommended number of reference subjects, we noted that Linnet's basic contribution to resolving this problem was in suggesting the ratio of the width of the 90 percent confidence interval for $\zeta_{0.975}$ to the width

---

[2] This formula does not require the two subgroup standard deviations to be of equal size, although they should both be smaller than the standard deviation σ of the combined group. Thus, if σ_g is the average subgroup standard deviation, then $h = (\sigma - \sigma_g)/\sigma$. It is assumed that the sample size n is large enough (> 50) to permit using the standard Normal deviate z and separate estimates of each standard deviation to test the observed difference. For large sample sizes, the test is essentially independent of the form of the distribution of values in either subgroup.

Table 3.1 z Values Required to Reduce Standard
Deviations by 10 Percent and 20 Percent

	z	
n	10% Reduction	20% Reduction
60	5.3	8.2
120	7.5	11.6
400	13.7	21.2
700	18.1	28.1
1000	21.7	33.5

Source: Harris and Boyd (1990), Table 1, p. 266.

of the 95 percent reference range as a criterion for determining
sample size. The idea of using the width of the 95 percent reference range as the basis for a numerical criterion has also been
suggested as a way of deciding whether or not separate reference ranges should be developed for particular subgroups of
the population. Sinton et al. (1986), in their large-scale study
of phosphorus, calcium, and alkaline phosphatase by age and
gender, proposed that separate reference ranges should not be
constructed unless the difference between subgroup means exceeded 25 percent of the 95 percent reference range for the combined group.

As an adjoint to their derivation of Equation (3.3), Harris
and Boyd (1990) proved the following relationship between z,
the standard Normal deviate, and p, the proportion of the 95
percent reference range represented by the difference between
two subgroup means:

$$z_p = 2p[2n/(1 - 4p^2)]^{1/2} \tag{3.4}$$

For example, when $n = 400$, and $p = .25$, $z_p = 16.3$. In
other words, using the value of p recommended by Sinton et
al., and with 400 subjects in each of two subgroups, the z-statis-
tic for the difference between the subgroup means would have

to exceed 16.3 before separate subgroup reference ranges would be recommended. Of course, this value far exceeds that required for statistical significance at, say, the 5 percent or 1 percent levels, but then so do the values given in Table 3.1. Equating the right-hand sides of Equations (3.3) and (3.4), we obtain the relation, $h = 1 - (1 - 4p^2)^{1/2}$, independent of sample size. Inserting the value $p = .25$, we calculate $h = 13.3$ percent. Thus, even when this rather stringent p value is satisfied, there is still not much reduction in variability.

3.3.1 Effects of Combined Reference Limits on Subgroups

Although the specific critical value (0.25) that Sinton and colleagues have proposed for the ratio (p) of the difference between subgroup means to the width of the reference range may be argued, their basic contribution has been to propose a different and, in our view, superior criterion than simply whether or not the difference between two subgroup means is statistically significant. For any critical value of this criterion, one may ask about the practical effects on individuals in a given subgroup when the critical value is not reached and the decision is made to use a single 95 percent reference range to represent the combined population.

In a purely statistical sense, the effect is to change for each subgroup the proportions of individuals above and below the reference limits from the nominal value of 2.5 percent for the entire group. This may be seen in Figure 3.4, which pictures two subgroup Normal distributions in different relations to each other, marking off the proportion of the tails of each distribution cut off by 95 percent limits based on the combined distributions.

In Figure 3.4a, the two subgroups have identical mean values, but differ in their standard deviations, one being 50 percent greater than the other. The result of using combined reference limits is that a much smaller proportion than 2.5 percent is excluded on either side of the narrower distribution, while a much larger proportion than 2.5 percent is outside the limit on either side of the wider distribution. Under any criterion that restricts

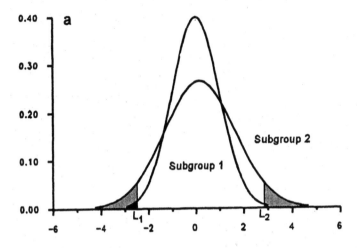

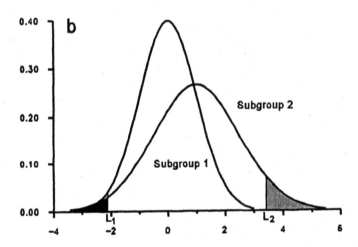

Fig. 3.4   Paired Normal distributions and 95 percent reference limits calculated from combined data base. The x-axis is in units of the standard deviation of subgroup 1 (σ_1). In both graphs, the SD of subgroup 2 (σ_2) is 50 percent larger than σ_1. (a) Means are equal ($\mu_1 = \mu_2$). (b) $\mu_2 = \mu_1 + \sigma_1$. (From Harris and Boyd, 1990, with permission.)

itself to the difference between the means with no regard for differences in the standard deviations, this situation may occur because separate reference ranges will never be established.

In Figure 3.4b, the two subgroups have different means as well as standard deviations. Here the proportions of individuals outside the reference limits not only are different for each subgroup but also within a subgroup are different for the upper reference limit than for the lower. None of these proportions is likely to equal 2.5 percent.

In both cases, assuming that these distributions represent healthy individuals, reference limits based on the combined data will produce specificities (probabilities of a false-positive decision) for each subgroup different from the expected 2.5 percent on each side. In choosing a criterion for establishing separate reference limits for subgroups, and deciding on a critical level for that criterion, we may reasonably ask about the effects of this decision on these specificities.

For example, in the case of the criterion proposed by Sinton et al., these effects can be determined numerically for two subgroups with the help of Equation (3.4) relating z, p, and n. Harris and Boyd (1990) carried out these calculations for $n = 120$ in each subgroup, assuming Normal distributions. Let us describe the procedures used and the results obtained.

First, we chose a series of z values: 0, 1, 2, 4, 6, 8. From Equation (3.4), for $n = 120$, these correspond, respectively, to the p values: 0, 0.032, 0.064, 0.095, 0.125, 0.18, 0.23, thus covering a range from a very permissive to a fairly stringent critical value for Sinton's ratio criterion. Next, we chose Normal subgroup distributions: first, as a base, the standard Normal distribution with mean $\mu = 0$ and standard deviation $\sigma = 1$. Other subgroup distributions for comparison with this base had standard deviations 1.0, 1.3, 1.5, and 2.0, respectively. Then, the means of these subgroup distributions were fixed by the selected values of their standard deviations and by the given values of z and n according to the standard Normal deviate test for the difference between two means, but substituting parameters for the usual statistics,

$$z = n^{1/2}(\mu_i - \mu)/(\sigma^2 + \sigma_i^2)^{1/2},$$

where μ_i and σ_i are the mean and standard deviation of the ith comparison subgroup and $\mu = 0$, $\sigma = 1$ are the parameters of the base subgroup. Therefore, $\mu_i = z[(1 + \sigma_i^2)/n]^{1/2}$. Note that the same value of μ_i for a larger sample size n would correspond to a larger value of z. This becomes important in relating the results obtained for $n = 120$ to corresponding critical values for larger sample sizes. Table 3.2 lists the values of these parameters.

Each of these 28 subgroups was paired with the standard Normal to form a combined distribution over two subgroups. Since the mixture of subgroups forms a nonNormal distribution, determining the effects of combined reference limits on

Table 3.2 Mean (μ_i) and Standard Deviation (σ_i) of Normal Subgroups for Comparison with Standard Normal ($\mu = 0$, $\sigma = 1$) at Listed Values of z and p and $n = 120$

z	p	σ_i	μ_i	z	p	σ_i	μ_i
0	0	1.0	0	4	0.125	1.0	0.52
		1.3	0			1.3	0.60
		1.5	0			1.5	0.66
		2.0	0			2.0	0.82
1	0.032	1.0	0.13	6	0.181	1.0	0.77
		1.3	0.15			1.3	0.90
		1.5	0.16			1.5	0.99
		2.0	0.20			2.0	1.22
2	0.064	1.0	0.26	8	0.229	1.0	1.03
		1.3	0.30			1.3	1.20
		1.5	0.33			1.5	1.32
		2.0	0.41			2.0	1.63
3	0.095	1.0	0.39				
		1.3	0.45				
		1.5	0.49				
		2.0	0.61				

the proportions excluded from each subgroup in the pair was done by simulation and estimation of the combined limits by the quantiles $Q_{0.025}$ and $Q_{0.975}$.[3] Random samples of 800 Normal deviates were drawn from each of the paired subgroups, so that the quantiles were based on 1600 values. To minimize the sampling variation in these quantile estimates, the random sampling process was repeated ten times for each pair. Thus, the final estimates were the means of ten replicate values.

These estimated reference limits for each combined group were then applied to the two subgroups, and the proportions of each subgroup falling outside the upper and lower reference limits were obtained using a standard algorithm for computing areas under the Normal curve (*Handbook of Mathematical Functions*, 1964, p. 932, Eq. 26.2.16). Results are presented in Figure 3.5. The top graph (a) shows how the proportion of the narrower (base) subgroup above the upper (97.5th) combined reference limit decreases as the wider subgroup ($\sigma_2 \geq 1$) moves farther to the right (increasing values of z). The bottom graph (b) shows how the proportion of the wider subgroup below the lower (2.5th) combined reference limit decreases under the same circumstances.

Let us focus on the curves for $\sigma_2 = 1.0$ and 1.3 since data from earlier studies (e.g. Wilding et al., 1972) and our own

---

[3] An alternative method, not involving simulation, might proceed as follows: The probability distribution of the mixture of two Normal subgroups may be written as $G(x) = p\phi_1(x) + (1 - p)\phi_2(x)$, where $\phi_1(x)$ and $\phi_2(x)$ are Normal distributions with means and standard deviations ($\mu = 0$, $\sigma = 1$) and ($\mu_2 = \mu_i = z[(1 + \sigma_i^2)/n]^{1/2}$, $\sigma_2 = \sigma_i$), respectively. In this case, $p = \frac{1}{2}$. Then, we want to find an upper reference limit, x_0 such that the integral of $G(x)$ from $-\infty$ to x_0 is equal to 0.975. This involves the weighted sum of two standard Normal integrals where the upper limit of the first is x_0, and the upper limit of the second is $y_0 = (x_0 - \mu_2)/\sigma_2$. We could not discover any direct solution for x_0; tedious trial and error seemed necessary for each pair of subgroups. Since smooth curves were not required for the final outcomes, but only accurate approximations, we decided on the simulation route described in the text.

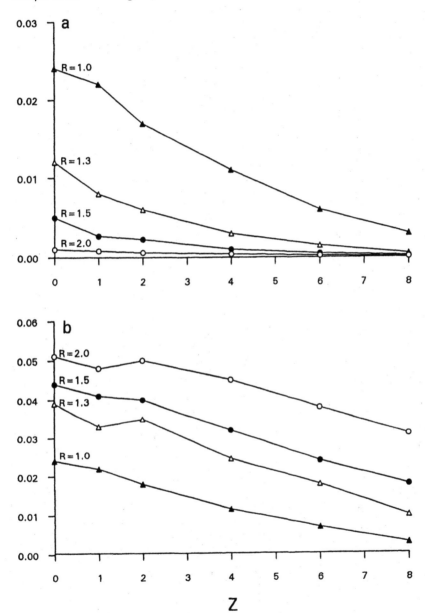

Fig. 3.5 (a) Proportion of the (narrower) subgroup 1 above the upper reference limit calculated from combined data base. (b) Proportion of the (wider) subgroup 2 below the lower combined reference limit. (From Harris and Boyd, 1990, with permission.)

experience indicated that even when mean values differ appreciably between subgroups, the standard deviations are seldom more than 30 percent apart and usually much closer. Suppose we argue that proportions expected to be around 2.5 percent should not fall below 1.0 percent. Interpolating roughly between the curves in Figure 3.5a for $\sigma_2 = 1.0$ and 1.3, we find that with respect to the upper reference limit, this condition is violated when z is greater than about 3. If, however, we argued that we would not be concerned until a subgroup proportion above the upper reference limit was only 0.5 percent or less, the critical value of z would rise to about 5. With respect to the lower reference limit, Figure 3.5b indicates a higher critical value of z for the 1.0 percent level, about 6, and even higher, about 8, for the 0.5 percent level. Note that these figures are based on a sample size of 120 in each subgroup.

Clearly, these results allow considerable latitude for choice. In our paper (Harris and Boyd, 1990) we gave greater emphasis to the upper reference limit as usually being of more practical concern and recommended $z = 3$ as a critical value (choosing the 1.0 percent barrier). This may be too permissive of separate subgroups, and a value of $z = 5$ might be a better compromise. Even with the higher value, given $n = 120$ per subgroup, the value of p, the ratio of the difference between subgroup means to the combined 95 percent reference range is 15.3 percent, considerably less than the 25 percent recommended by Sinton et al.

If we fix Sinton's ratio p at a selected point, say p_0, then Equation (3.4) provides a relationship between the critical value of z at p_0 for a given sample size n and the critical value of z at p_0 for any other sample size. We denote these critical values by $z_n^*(p_0)$. Suppose we set $p_0 = 0.153$, that is, $z_{120}^*(0.153) = 5.0$. Then this value of p_0 will be maintained for any sample size if we calculate the critical value at that sample size as

$$z_n^*(p_0 = 0.153) = 5(n/120)^{1/2}. \tag{3.5}$$

Thus, for example, if $n = 400$ in each subgroup, $z_{400}^*(p_0 = 0.153)$

= 9.13. Figure 3.6 graphs Equation (3.5) for values of n from 100 to 1200. There is additional information to be gained from the results shown in Figure 3.5. Recall that σ_2 is actually the ratio of the two subgroup standard deviations in any pair since the standard deviation of the base subgroup is unity. We see from Figure 3.5a that when $\sigma_2 \geq 1.5$, the proportion of the narrower subgroup above the upper reference limit is less than 0.5 percent *regardless of the difference between subgroup means*. What is happening, as we can judge from Figure 3.4, is that when the ratio of standard deviations equals or exceeds 1.5, the wider subgroup tends to completely cover the narrower distribution, at least until the former moves sufficiently far to the right (a z value of at least 4 at a sample size of 120 per subgroup). Harris and Boyd (1990) recommended that if the ratio of subgroup standard deviations equals or exceeds 1.5,

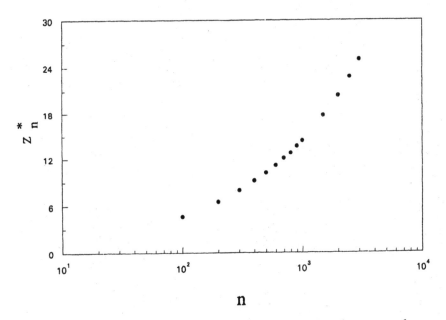

Fig. 3.6 Critical value of z for sample size n in each subgroup, calculated from Equation (3.5).

then separate reference ranges should be calculated regardless of whether the means are significantly different statistically.

3.3.2 Examples

Table 3.3 presents means and standard deviations of high-density lipoproteins and calcium measured in blood samples collected from three successive classes of medical students at the University of Virginia during 1987 and 1988 (Harris and Boyd, 1990). These statistics were derived from 120 men and 120 women between 20 and 30 years of age. Also shown are the statistics of the combined group and the z values for the differences between subgroup means. Within each sex, the distributions were very close to Normal. The ratios of the mean differences to the combined parametric reference ranges were close to those predicted from Equation (3.4). This formula is essentially nonparametric and should be valid for moderately skewed as well as symmetric distributions.

For both analytes, the z values exceeded 5. In fact, gender-related differences in these analytes at young adult ages are well known although they have not been recognized in routine laboratory reports. The 95 percent reference range for the combined calcium data was 90.4 to 103.2 g/L. The data showed that none of the women exceeded the upper limit, and none of the men were below the lower limit.

Table 3.3 Means, Standard Deviations, and z values of HDL (g/L) and Calcium (g/L) in Medical Students: 120 Men and 120 Women

Analyte	Means			Standard deviations			z
	Men	Women	Comb.	Men	Women	Comb.	
HDL	453	560	506.5	92.9	100.8	110.7	8.6
Calcium	98.0	95.7	96.8	3.1	2.9	3.2	5.8

Another example concerns differences in creatine kinase (CK) among racial and gender subgroups. Such differences were confirmed in data collected and interpreted by Wong et al. (1983) in a study of over 1500 apparently healthy employees at a medical center in Los Angeles. These data were reexamined by Harris et al. (1991) to assess the application of Harris and Boyd's simulation study and the ratio criterion proposed by Sinton et al.

Wong et al. found three categories of CK levels according to race–gender groups: high CK, seen in black men; intermediate CK, occurring in Hispanic, Asian and white men and black women; and low CK, in Asian, Hispanic, and white women. Table 3.4 presents the sample sizes, means, and standard deviations of log CK within each category along with 95 percent parametric reference ranges based on the log transform.

The z values associated with differences between these means were 11.6 comparing the high and intermediate categories, and 17.0 comparing the intermediate and low categories. The sample sizes in the latter two categories were about the same, averaging 656, and the z value of 17.0 is far above the critical value for this sample size according to Figure 3.6 ($z^* = 11.7$). The sample sizes in the high and intermediate categories were quite different, but using the average sample size, the observed z substantially exceeds the critical value of $z^* = 9.5$.

Table 3.4 Statistics for log CK and 95 Percent Reference Ranges in High, Intermediate, and Low Categories

Category	n	log CK Mean	SD	95% Reference ranges (U/L), parametric
High	195	2.231	0.270	50–574
Intermediate	668	1.984	0.229	34–270
Low	645	1.785	0.195	25–147

Source: Harris et al. (1991), Table 2, p. 1581.

The classification by Wong et al. of CK into three racial–gender categories satisfies the criteria for separate reference ranges based on Harris and Boyd's simulation studies. To see what values of Sinton's ratio criterion this classification represents, we may use Equation (3.4), inserting the observed values of z, the average sample sizes, and solving for p in each case. Results are 0.18 for the high versus intermediate classification and 0.21 for the intermediate versus low category. Although these values are less than that recommended by Sinton et al. for establishing separate reference ranges, it seems evident that these separate categories for creatine kinase are justified.

3.3.3 More Than Two Subgroups

The criteria discussed above for separate reference ranges have been based on theory and simulations of only two subgroups. When more than two subgroups are suggested by the data, the question of what statistical criteria should be satisfied may be more difficult to resolve. In the case of three categories, the simplest procedure would be to perform two separate z-tests, as was done for the creatine kinase data of Wong et al.

Another alternative, particularly when more than three categories are involved, is to start by carrying out an analysis of variance of all results together, using a generalized least squares program if necessary to take account of varying numbers of subjects in each subgroup. A significant F-test from this analysis should then be followed by simultaneous comparison of paired means, preferably, in our opinion, the Tukey test, which controls all such comparisons at the 0.05 probability level while maintaining a high probability of detecting real differences between pairs. Any pair of means whose difference is statistically significant should then be reexamined against the more stringent z^* critical levels suggested earlier.

3.3.4 Application to the Design of a Reference Value Study

If there is good reason to expect that separate reference ranges will be justifiable and clinically useful for an analyte about to be measured in a given population, then one would want to allow, if possible, for a sufficient number of reference subjects *within each subgroup*. Selection of this number might be guided by Figures 3.2 and 3.3, for example. As mentioned earlier, this in itself would require information about coefficients of variation gained from early data or a separate pilot study. These same data would provide material for preliminary z-tests or analysis of variance among subgroup means. The number of subjects should, if possible, be approximately the same for each subgroup. Results of these analyses could be compared with the critical value of z for the average sample size per subgroup. If statistical justification for separate reference ranges appears to be present, the study should continue sampling subjects to reach the desired number within each subgroup.

3.4 OUTLIERS

The question of whether or not to exclude outlying observations arises from a general concern with the homogeneity of reference sets. The name *outliers* implies that individual measurements have been ordered by size and their distribution displayed graphically. Sorting and display of data is relatively easy to carry out with modern computing equipment, and many ways have been developed to illustrate the variation contained in a set of observations (e.g., Chambers et al., 1983). Indeed, inspecting the distribution of individual results, at least in tabular form and preferably graphically, is essential before embarking on any statistical analysis to derive reference ranges. This is true even if the statistical method employed is robust against outliers, that is, more or less impervious to the effects of extreme values.

We define outliers not merely as the least or greatest of a set of observations, but as data points, either singly or in a group, that lie noticeably distant from their closest neighbors. First of all, we want to account for these extreme values, if possible. Are they traceable to outright blunders in biochemical analysis or in recording results? Do they reflect a short-term episode of unusual bias in the analytical procedure that would also be apparent in quality control samples? In this case, unless known mistakes can be corrected, attempts to adjust the numbers are probably ill-advised, and the offending data should be discarded. Do the outliers represent subjects with unusual characteristics (e.g., violating some pre-analytical rules of behavior, such as no heavy exercise before sampling) or, more importantly, some special demographic trait that distinguishes these subjects from the others? Such observations should be eliminated from the current reference set but may signal the need for testing additional subjects with the same demographic characteristic.

If no reason can be found to explain extreme results, and they occur on the long tail of a skewed distribution, they should probably be retained. As Barnett and Lewis (1994) and others have pointed out, apparently aberrant extreme values may in fact be the result of chance selection from an asymmetric distribution underlying all the observations. A transformation process might bring all the observations into an approximately Normal form or at least clearly separate some or all of the original outliers from the Normal distribution of the rest of the data on the transformed scale. Then, various options exist either to test the heterogeneity of the remaining outliers or to obtain robust estimators of the mean and standard deviation of the assumed Normal distribution in spite of these outliers so that reliable estimators of the reference limits can be derived. We describe briefly some of these methods below.

Most of the techniques for dealing with outliers in clinical chemistry have been developed in the context of internal or external quality control studies where Normal distributions are the rule. A common procedure has been to calculate the mean and standard deviation of all the observations and then discard those values that fall outside the mean plus or minus some multiple of the standard deviation. For example, Burnett (1975) suggested the multiple 3.52 for 120 observations and gives a table of multiplers for other sample sizes, based on a modification of a method proposed by Natrella (1963, p. 17-4). After one or more outliers have been deleted, the process is repeated, computing a new mean and standard deviation each time, until no further outliers are found. If the great majority of the observations are distributed symmetrically with a relatively small standard deviation, the true standard deviation may at first be overestimated and outliers included that should not be. However, these are likely to be caught in the next iteration. A recent study by Thienpont et al. (1987), based on results of external quality control surveys in which the bulk of reported results were approximately Normally distributed, also proposed a set of multipliers varying with sample size, quite similar to Burnett's in the range of 60–400 observations.

Again in the context of quality control surveys, and assuming an underlying Normal distribution, Healy (1979) described a symmetric "trimming" procedure to obtain a robust estimate of the standard deviation. A small percentage of the observations (say, 2–3 percent) are cut off each end. The standard deviation is then estimated from the formula

$$\sigma = b_p \sum_{i=1}^{k} \frac{(2i - k - 1)x_{(i)}}{k(k - \frac{1}{2})}, \tag{3.6}$$

where k denotes the number of observations left after trimming, $x_{(i)}$ is the ith order statistic in the trimmed sample, and b_p is an "unbiasing factor" depending on the proportion p of observations remaining. Healy gives a table of b_p for p from 0.50 to 0.98, but recommends trimming no more than 10 percent of the sample. Since this proportion will almost certainly include all apparent outliers, the net effect of their deviations may be assessed without worry that retaining or deleting any particular outlier will influence the estimated standard deviation.

Barnett and Lewis (1994) discuss a wide variety of statistical techniques for testing the atypicality of outlying observations. One general class of tests due to Dixon (1953) computes ratios D/R, where, for example, D is the difference between the extreme observation and its nearest neighbor, and R is the range of all observations. Unfortunately, significance points for such ratios have been computed only for sample sizes of 30 or less.

The theory assumes that the underlying distribution, exclusive of contaminating data points, is Normal, although Barnett and Lewis discuss the Dixon class and other ratio criteria for asymmetric distributions as well.

Reed et al. (1971) proposed use of the particular Dixon ratio mentioned above for cross-sectional reference data. They suggested that if this ratio exceeds $\frac{1}{3}$, the outlier should be deleted. This is a highly conservative criterion, with a probability of less than 1 percent of erroneously eliminating an observation that belongs to the same (Normal) distribution as the other data points. Since most observed cross-sectional distributions do not follow the Normal form, this degree of conservatism may be warranted if the $\frac{1}{3}$ rule is applied to the original observations but not if it is applied to transformed observations that are approximately Normally distributed. Another problem arises when more than one outlier is present on the same side of the distribution, causing the D/R rule to fail and masking the presence of less extreme values. In such a case, the D/R rule might be applied to the least extreme outlier. Alternatively, a test called a "block" procedure, which considers all the outliers together, might be applied; examples are given in Barnett and Lewis (1994).

Finally, we mention a nonparametric technique suggested by Tukey (1977) that uses the sample "interquartile distance," $H = Q_{0.75} - Q_{0.25}$. Tukey defines a "lower outer fence," LOF $= Q_{0.25} - 3.0(H)$, a "lower inner fence," LIF $= Q_{0.25} - 1.5(H)$, an "upper outer fence," UOF $= Q_{0.75} + 3.0(H)$, and an "upper inner fence," UIF $= Q_{0.75} + 1.5(H)$. Observations outside the outer fences are "far out"; those between inner and outer fences are simply "outside." Under a Normal distribution, $H = 1.35\sigma$, so that UOF and LOF are equal to $\mu \pm 4.725\sigma$, while UIF and LIF are $\mu \pm 2.70\sigma$. One might argue, then, that data values beyond the outer fences should be deleted, while those between outer and inner fences should be retained unless we have other information about specific observations that suggests they be rejected. Tukey himself was silent on the question of keeping or rejecting outliers.

Clearly, there are many ways of testing the acceptability of outlying observations. An advantage of the parametric method of estimating reference limits is that if it succeeds in converting at least the great majority of reference values to Normal form, then a trimming procedure like Healy's may be applied to obtain a robust estimate of the standard deviation on the transformed scale without the need to decide on individual outliers. On the other hand, the nonparametric bootstrap estimator of Harrell and Davis is also robust against outlying observations because it is a weighted average of all the sample quantiles. The single-quantile estimator $Q_{0.025}$ or $Q_{0.975}$ in a sample of size 100 or so is little affected by the actual values of one or two extreme results so long as they remain part of the data. However, these estimators may be greatly affected by a decision to delete extremal values.

3.5 TRANSFERENCE OF REFERENCE RANGES

Manufacturers of devices for measuring the concentrations of biochemical analytes in blood are required by law in the United States to determine 95 percent reference ranges using these devices. These ranges are then printed in the material accompanying the instruments when they are received by user laboratories. Presumably, the distribution of test values found for individual reference subjects is also available on request, but such requests are apparently very rarely made.

Users of these devices are now by law required to validate these manufacturers' ranges in their own laboratories. The question of the number of reference subjects needed to estimate reference ranges thus becomes of importance to the entire universe of clinical laboratories. Sample sizes that are not unreasonable for large manufacturers are imposssible for small user laboratories and might be very difficult even for clinical laboratories in large teaching hospitals. A possible solution for laboratories in the latter category (or for groups of laboratories within a given geographic region) would be to develop a large roster of randomly selected, consenting reference subjects in the area, draw a single blood specimen from each, and maintain those specimens (or the sera) under very deep freeze. Then, minute volumes can be drawn from each sample whenever reference ranges are required for newly received analytical devices. The analyses would be performed by a selected user laboratory in the area and results accepted by all area users of that device. This assumes, of course, that strict adherence to the same analytical procedure (usually that recommended by the manufacturer) would be followed in practice by all area laboratories.

Even with such a resource available, user laboratories would wish to compare the ranges obtained with those published by the manufacturer. For this purpose, one may apply the criteria recommended in Section 3.3.1 for determining whether two separate ranges should be maintained—in this case, the manufacturer's and the users'. The manufacturer would have to supply at least the mean, standard deviation and sample size that was employed along with information about any transformations of data. Indeed, such information should be made available with the printed material accompanying the device as distributed.

Another possible approach for small laboratories that wish to validate manufacturers' reference ranges independently is to obtain and analyze specimens from, say, 20 apparently healthy individuals believed to be representative of their general practice. From simple binomial theory, the probability that more than 2 out of 20 results would lie outside the manufacturer's reference range, when the laboratory's true 95 percent range was identical, is approximately 7.5 percent. This calculation assumes that the manufacturer's reference range is based on at least 100 subjects (see Van Der Meulen et al., 1994). If more than two results fall outside the published range, the laboratory should repeat the trial with another 20 reference subjects. Failure again to find at least 18 results within the range should lead to a review of the analytic procedure actually followed by the user, but might imply a patient population substantially different biologically from that sampled by the manufacturer. In this case, separate ranges may be necessary, based on at least 60 individuals.

APPENDIX 3.1 BASIC PROGRAM FOR SAMPLE SIZES UNDER POWER TRANSFORM

```
5 REM PROGR. FOR SAMPLE SIZES UNDER POWER TRANSFORM Y=X^m

10 REM L=1/m

20 REM C IS THE C.V. OF TRANSFORMED DATA

30 REM R IS THE RATIO OF 90% CONF. INTERVAL FOR UPPER

40 REM REF. LIMIT TO 95% REF. RANGE

50 REM IF R IS NOT EQUAL TO 0.2 CHANGE STATEMENT 60

55 OPEN "LPT1:" FOR OUTPUT AS #1

60 R=.2

70 FOR L=2 TO 4

80 FOR C=.2 TO 1 STEP .2

90 A=1+1.96*C

100 B=2.811*C

110 A1=1-1.96*C

120 D=A^L-A1^L

130 D=D*R

140 IF L=3 GO TO 180

150 IF L=4 GO TO 200

160 T=4*A*B

170 GO TO 220

180 T=6*A^2*B

190 GO TO 220
```

```
200 T=8*A^3*B
220 N=(T/D)^2
230 PRINT #1, "L=",L,"C=",C,"N=",N
240 NEXT C
250 NEXT L
300 END
```

APPENDIX 3.2 SAMPLE SIZES FOR LOGNORMAL DISTRIBUTIONS

Back-transforming $y = \log_e x$ to the original (x) scale requires exponentiating the Normal estimators and their large-sample confidence limits. The 90 percent confidence interval for the upper 95 percent reference limit becomes

$$\exp(\bar{y} + 1.96 s_y + 2.811 s_y/n^{1/2}) - \exp(\bar{y} + 1.96 s_y - 2.811 s_y/n^{1/2}$$
$$= \exp(\bar{y} + 1.96 s_y)[\exp(2.811 s_y/n^{1/2}) - \exp(-2.811 s_y/n^{1/2})],$$

while the 95 percent reference range on the original scale is

$$\exp(\bar{y})[\exp(1.96 s_y) - \exp(-1.96 s_y)],$$

where $\bar{y}$ and s_y are the mean and SD, respectively, of the logarithms. Then the ratio of the confidence interval to the reference range becomes

$$R = \frac{\exp(2.811 s_y/n^{1/2}) - \exp(-2.811 s_y/n^{1/2})}{1 - \exp(-3.92 s_y)}$$

$$= \frac{2 \sinh(2.811 s_y/n^{1/2})}{1 - \exp(-3.92 s_y)},$$

or $\sinh(2.811 s_y/n^{1/2}) = (R/2)[1 - \exp(-3.92 s_y)$, where $\sinh(t)$ denotes the hyperbolic sine of t.

Now, under the logNormal distribution, the SD of $y = \log_e x$ is related to the CV of x according to the formula, $s_y =$

$[\log_e(1 + C_x^2)]^{1/2}$. For values of C_x from 0.2 to 3.0, s_y will vary from 0.198 to 1.517, and the quantity $(R/2)[1 - \exp(-3.92s_y)]$ when $R = 0.2$ will vary from 0.0540 to 0.0996. For such small values, $\sinh(t)$ and t itself are virtually equal; therefore, we may write $2.811s_y/n^{1/2} = (R/2)[1 - \exp(-3.96s_y)]$. From this equation, setting $R = 0.2$ and using the relation between s_y and C_x, we calculated the graph of n versus C_x shown in Figure 3.3.

4

MULTIVARIATE REFERENCE REGIONS AND INDICES

4.1 INTRODUCTION

In theory, the subject of multivariate reference regions (MRRs) for biochemical analytes follows naturally after univariate reference limits. In practice, however, the MRR remains a statistical curiosity to the great majority of clinical chemists and clinicians and has little or no use in present-day clinical practice. A rare exception like the trivariate region of thyroid tests developed by Kägedal et al. (1978, 1982) seems only to prove the rule.

Yet MRRs are not new to the clinical laboratory literature, going back more than 20 years to Grams et al. (1972) and Winkel et al. (1972). Many reviews of biochemical data in patients and healthy subjects (e.g., Winkel et al., 1972; Rehpenning et al., 1979; Kägedal et al., 1982; Boyd and Lacher, 1982) as well as simulation studies (e.g., Harris, 1981) have demonstrated that the use of MRRs instead of multiple univariate ranges can greatly reduce the risk of false-positive diagnosis. Moreover, clinical laboratories routinely perform a variety of organ-specific test panels, each of which includes multiple laboratory analytes. This should be fertile ground for the development and use of MRRs appropriate for different organ-specific pathologies.

How then explain the neglect of these potentially useful statistical tools? To find some answers to this question, Durbridge (1983) conducted the following experiment. First, he chose a panel of six biochemical tests (albumin, globulin, bilirubin, alkaline phosphatase, lactate dehydrogenase and aspartate aminotransferase), rather oriented toward hepatobiliary problems. Then, based on results from 223 apparently healthy laboratory staff workers, he computed a multivariate reference index (see below) for each reference subject and determined the 95 percent sample quantile. This implied that about 95 percent of patients who resemble the reference subjects in these six tests should present index values less than (or equal to) the 95 percent quantile, or less than unity if divided by the 95 percent quantile.

Durbridge designated this ratio an STSS ("six-test signal strength") and added the STSS value to the laboratory report for each patient whose physician had ordered this panel of tests during a 4-month period. At the beginning of the trial, clinicians were notified that the STSS represented the "degree of abnormality overall," and were presented with a table to help them interpret the reported value. Thus, STSS values from zero to unity were called "physiological"; 1–4, "not unusual for inpatients"; 4–10, "moderate"; 10–20, "strong"; and >20, "gross abnormality." These grades were based on an empirical distribution of STSS values determined earlier for hospital patients. Of course, results of the separate biochemical tests and their 95 percent reference ranges were also included.

Durbridge reported that roughly a third of the 129 clinicians interviewed at the end of the study found the STSS value of no use to them and disregarded it, another third believed it of some help, while the final group felt they needed more experience with the index before drawing any conclusion about its usefulness. Among many reasons offered for ignoring the index were the following: (1) the cause of a high STSS (presumably just one or two of the six tests) was already obvious to the physician, so the combined index provided no additional information and was distracting; (2) although the STSS was high, nothing strikingly abnormal was seen in the individual tests, and therefore the index was ignored; (3) clinicians expert in their particular fields had already selected the specific tests they desired, and saw no advantage in combining these with others they were not interested in; (4) clinicians tend to be concerned only with high values of the tests included, so a high index value due to an unusually low result for one or two of the tests would be deemed of no clinical significance. On the other hand, physicians who reported the multivariate index as helpful remarked that a high value caused them to look more carefully at the individual test values and detect an abnormal test that might otherwise have been overlooked.

As indicated earlier, the most distinctive feature of an MRR is its ability to submerge the sporadic "false-positive" result of a single test and thereby save the cost of needless follow-up laboratory testing and clinical investigation. To evaluate the real impact of this advantage in clinical practice, a more elaborate randomized controlled study would be required including patients whose laboratory reports did not contain the multivariate index. Nevertheless, Durbridge's experiment clarified another important aspect of the use of MRRs or indices based on them. As the author pointed out, such indices will not be readily accepted unless clinicians are informed by the laboratory of the possible interpretations of any abnormal index value contained in the patient's laboratory report. This is particularly true when the individual tests all appear to be within their reference ranges.

This type of disagreement between the multivariate index and the separate test results is infrequent, but does occur; it was noted by Healy (1969) many years ago. In their study of both simulated and real biochemical test data, Harris et al. (1982) found that when three analytes were included in a 95 percent MRR, about 1.5 percent of combined sets fell outside the MRR and each separate analyte appeared within its own 95 percent reference range. Despite this low frequency overall, such discrepancies accounted for about one-quarter of all the abnormal multivariate results. The reason usually lies in the correlation between a particular pair of analytes. The MRR takes all such pairwise correlations into account, and this is its fundamental strength vis-à-vis separate reference ranges. On occasion, however, a set of results will contain observations for two analytes in just the opposite direction from that expected by the overall correlation for that pair, producing a multivariate abnormality not reflected in the separate constituents.

Interestingly, one kind of hybrid univariate has long been accepted as part of routine practice in the clinical laboratory: the ratio of two physiologically related constituents. An example is the ratio of urea nitrogen (BUN) to serum creatinine (SCr) as a means of differential diagnosis among renal diseases or distinguishing between renal and other problems. A high BUN/SCr ratio (> 20) may indicate gastrointestinal bleeding, dehydration or early acute glomerulonephritis, whereas a low ratio (< 10) may indicate acute tubular nephrosis or simply the effect of severe exercise before blood drawing. Although such ratios have solid bases in physiology and have often proved clinically useful, it is possible that they might beneficially be supplemented by multivariate indices that include three or four related variables. We explore this possibility in analyzing data on BUN, SCr, and uric acid (UA) in Section 4.6.

Even if the MRR or a related multivariate index becomes more popular than it seems to be today, it will probably almost always be computed from measurements in healthy subjects rather than ill patients, just as is the case for univariate reference limits. However, another multivariate technique, discriminant function analysis (DA), has been used for many years to test selected biochemical analytes for their abilities to distinguish among related disease processes—that is, to aid the clinician in differential diagnosis. Although closely related statistically to MRRs, and probably the multivariate statistical methodology best known to clinical chemists, DA lies outside the scope of this book. The literature on the subject is vast, but, in our view, the best single source of information about DA for clinical chemists is the recent review by Solberg (1985).

MRRs in practical use are almost always derived from the assumption that the selected set of variate values are jointly distributed in a multivariate Normal distribution. This assumption is not essential to the development of a multivariate index; however, the form of the multivariate Normal distribution leads directly to a powerful index, the Mahalanobis *distance function*.

4.2 THE BIVARIATE NORMAL DISTRIBUTION

The simplest MRR is that obtained from the joint distribution of two variables, so we take the bivariate Normal distribution as our starting point. However, to help understand the bivariate reference region, we refer to the univariate Normal density function:

$$f(x) = \text{pr}(x) = (\sqrt{2\pi}\, \sigma)^{-1} \exp\{-\tfrac{1}{2}[(x - \mu)/\sigma]^2\},$$

with mean μ and standard deviation σ, pictured in Figure 4.1.

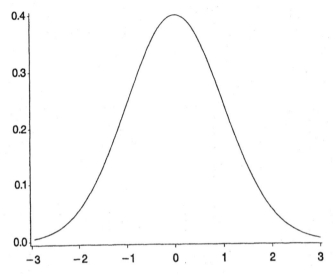

Fig. 4.1 Univariate Normal probability density function. (Standardized: $\rho = 0$, $\sigma = 1$.)

Suppose we add to this picture a horizontal line just touching the curve at its peak ($x = \mu$). Now imagine this line slowly descending toward the x-axis through a series of stops and starts. At any stop in its descent, the line will cut the Normal curve at two points equidistant from the mean. Perpendiculars from these points to the x-axis define a segment of the axis. The area under the curve above this segment represents that proportion of the population of values lying within the segment. The length of the segment is then the $100p$ percent reference range for a Normally distributed biochemical analyte.

The joint Normal distribution of two variables, say x_1 and x_2, is given by the formula

$$f(x_1, x_2) = (2\pi\sigma_1\sigma_2 \sqrt{1 - \rho_{12}^2})^{-1}$$
$$\cdot \exp\{[-\tfrac{1}{2}(1 - \rho^2)^{-1}]([(x_1 - \mu_1)/\sigma_1]^2 \qquad (4.1)$$
$$+ [(x_2 - \mu_2)/\sigma_2]^2 - 2\rho_{12}[(x_1 - \mu_1)(x_2 - \mu_2)/\sigma_1\sigma_2])\},$$

where μ_1, μ_2, σ_1, and σ_2 are the means and standard deviations of x_1 and x_2, and ρ_{12} is the correlation between the variables. This formula is pictured in Figure 4.2.

Now consider a plane parallel to the x_1, x_2 plane starting at the peak of this bell-shaped surface ($x_1 = \mu_1$, $x_2 = \mu_2$) and slowly descending with stops and starts towards the x_1, x_2 plane. At each stop, it will define an elliptical cross section of the bivariate surface that contains a specific proportion p of all pairs of values x_1, x_2, depending on the stopping point along the axis $f(x_1, x_2)$. As the descending plane moves closer to the x_1, x_2 plane, the areas of the ellipses increase, each containing a larger proportion of values than the preceding ones. Projecting all of them to the x_1, x_2 plane, they form a set of concentric ellipses.

Each of these ellipses is the boundary of a region containing those pairs x_1, x_2 that, when inserted into the right-hand side of Equation (4.1), yield values of $f(x_1, x_2)$ less than or equal to some constant, say c_p. When the values represent measure-

$f(x_1, x_2)$

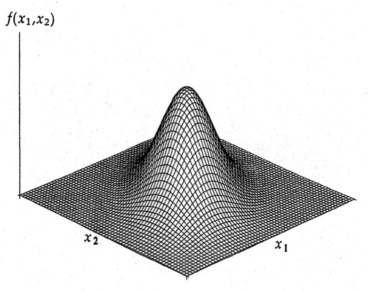

Fig. 4.2 Bivariate Normal probability density function.

ments of two biochemical analytes, we presume that each pair is contributed by a different individual, the ith subject.

Since the only random variables in (4.1) are those terms in the exponential, an equivalent region, the bivariate reference region, may be defined by the inequality

$$(1 - \rho_{12}^2)^{-1}\{(x_1 - \mu_1)^2/\sigma_1^2 + (x_2 - \mu_2)^2/\sigma_2^2$$
$$- 2\rho_{12}(x_1 - \mu_1)(x_2 - \mu_2)/\sigma_1\sigma_2\} \le K_p, \tag{4.2}$$

where K_p is another constant.

We need to determine K_p so that those x_1, x_2 pairs that define the boundary of this region may be calculated. This is most easily done by, first, expressing the left-hand side of (4.2) in terms of the standardized variables, $z_1 = (x_1 - \mu_1)/\sigma_1$, and $z_2 = (x_2 - \mu_2)/\sigma_2$, so that

$$(1 - \rho_{12}^2)^{-1}(z_1^2 + z_2^2 - 2\rho_{12}z_1z_2) \le K_p. \tag{4.3}$$

Next, z_1 and z_2 are converted to independent variables, say, u_1 and u_2, through the linear transforms

$$u_1 = [2(1 + \rho_{12})]^{-1/2}(z_1 + z_2),$$
$$u_2 = [2(1 - \rho_{12})]^{-1/2}(z_1 - z_2), \tag{4.4}$$

so that now

$$u_1^2 + u_2^2 \le K_p. \tag{4.5}$$

Just as z_1 and z_2 are Normally distributed, so u_1 and u_2 are also Normal by the reproductive property of this distribution. It is a simple exercise to show that u_1 and u_2 have zero means, unit standard deviations and zero covariance.

These transforms are the simplest examples of converting a set of dependent variables to independent variables through the eigenvalues and eigenvectors of the covariance matrix or, as in this case, the correlation matrix (defined later). A brief review of these quantities is given in Appendix 4.1.1. The general theory may be found in texts of multivariate analysis or factor analysis (e.g., by Johnson and Wichern, 1988).

Since u_1 and u_2 are independent Normally distributed variables with zero means and unit standard deviations, the sum of their squares is distributed in a chi-square distribution with two degrees of freedom. Therefore, the $(100p)$ percent bivariate Normal reference region contains all pairs of values x_1, x_2 for which the left-hand side of Equation (4.2), denoted, say, by $\delta_2{}^2$, satisfies the inequality

$$\delta_2{}^2 \leq \chi^2_{2,p}, \tag{4.6}$$

where the right-hand side is the $(100p)th$ percentile of the chi-square distribution with two degrees of freedom. For example, a 95 percent bivariate Normal reference region contains those pairs x_1, x_2 for which $\delta_2{}^2 \leq 5.991$. The shape and orientation of these reference regions with respect to the x_1, x_2 plane depends on the standard deviations σ_1, σ_2 and the correlation ρ_{12}, as indicated in Figure 4.3.

To compute the reference region bounded by $\chi^2_{2,p}$, the population parameters μ_1, μ_2, σ_1, σ_2, and ρ_{12} must be known. In practice, of course, they are unknown and must be estimated from a cross-sectional sample of individuals assumed representative of the desired population. However, using the sample values $\bar{x}_1$, $\bar{x}_2$, s_1, s_2, and r_{12} to compute an estimate $D_2{}^2$ of $\delta_2{}^2$, one can no longer be certain that the region defined by $D_2{}^2 \leq \chi^2_{2,p}$ contains $100p$ percent of the population of paired values x_1, x_2.

Under these circumstances, the reference region becomes a *tolerance region*, that is, a region that has only a probability, say γ, of containing $100p$ percent of the population of bivariate measurements. In discussing this point, Albert and Harris (1987, p. 58) recommended that the most appropriate tolerance region for clinical use would be that for which $\gamma = 0.50$. This characterizes a region that, *on the average*, contains exactly $100p$ percent of the population. As Chew (1966) pointed out, the advantage of such a region is that it represents a *prediction region*

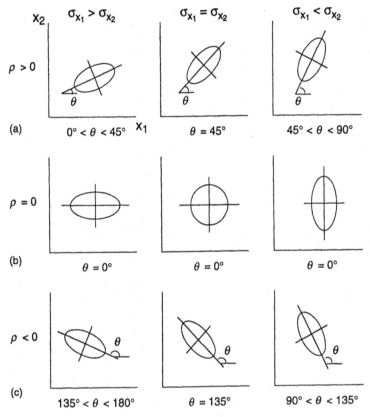

Fig. 4.3 Constant probability regions of bivariate Normal distributions. (From Johnson and Kotz, 1972.)

that may be used to evaluate the abnormality of a single set of observations from an individual. This is the purpose that multivariate reference regions would indeed serve in clinical laboratory practice. In the bivariate case, such a reference region would contain those points satisfying the inequality,

$$D_2^2 \leq 2(n^2 - 1)F(p; 2, n - 2)/n(n - 2), \tag{4.7}$$

where n is the sample size and $F(p; 2, n - 2)$ denotes the

$(100p)$th percentile of the F-distribution for 2 and $n - 2$ degrees of freedom. For large sample sizes, $(n^2 - 1)/n$, may be replaced by n. Then, a 95 percent bivariate reference region, based on, say 200 observations of x_1, x_2 would be bounded by the ellipse $D_2^2 = 6.10$. For sample sizes this large, there is little difference between this multivariate prediction region and the MPR defined by $\chi_{2,0.95}^2 = 5.991$.

4.3 MULTIVARIATE REGIONS AND INDICES

The theory underlying the bivariate Normal reference region extends straightforwardly to the MRR for more than two variables, but expression in compact form requires the use of matrix notation, and full understanding requires familiarity with matrix operations. We provide here no more than the bare minimum needed to describe an MRR.

Let a set of measurements on k variables be denoted by the column vector

$$
\mathbf{x} = \begin{bmatrix} x_1 \\ x_2 \\ \vdots \\ x_k \end{bmatrix}
$$

or the row vector $\mathbf{x}' = [x_1, x_2, \ldots, x_k]$, where the prime indicates the operation of transposing a column to a row. The vector of population means may then be written $\boldsymbol{\mu}' = [\mu_1, \mu_2, \ldots, \mu_k]$, and similarly, the vector of means from a sample of observation vectors $\mathbf{x}$ would be $\bar{\mathbf{x}}' = [\bar{x}_1, \bar{x}_2, \ldots, \bar{x}_k]$.

The matrix of population variances and covariances is usually expressed in the form

$$
\boldsymbol{\Sigma} = \begin{bmatrix} \sigma_{11} & \sigma_{12} & \cdots & \sigma_{1k} \\ \sigma_{21} & \sigma_{22} & \cdots & \sigma_{2k} \\ \vdots & \vdots & & \vdots \\ \sigma_{k1} & \sigma_{k2} & \cdots & \sigma_{kk} \end{bmatrix},
$$

where the variances appear along the main diagonal and the covariances in the off-diagonal positions. In the positional notation of matrices, the first subscript refers to the row of the element and the second to the column. Thus, σ_{ii} denotes the variance of the ith variable ($i = 1, \ldots, k$), and σ_{ij} ($i \neq j$), the covariance of the ith and jth variables ($\sigma_{ij} = \rho_{ij}\sqrt{\sigma_{ii}\sigma_{jj}}$). Similarly, the sample variances and covariances are expressed in matrix form as

$$
\mathbf{S} = \begin{bmatrix}
s_{11} & s_{12} & \cdots & s_{1k} \\
s_{21} & s_{22} & \cdots & s_{2k} \\
\vdots & \vdots & & \vdots \\
s_{k1} & s_{k2} & \cdots & s_{kk}
\end{bmatrix}.
$$

Both $\boldsymbol{\Sigma}$ and $\mathbf{S}$ are square $k \times k$ matrices (equal number of rows and columns) and symmetric (the elements above the main diagonal are equal to elements in the transposed position below the main diagonal). The vectors $\boldsymbol{\mu}'$ and $\bar{\mathbf{x}}'$ are $1 \times k$ matrices: one row and k columns. The correlation matrix is symmetric and defined as

$$
\boldsymbol{\rho} = \begin{bmatrix}
1 & \rho_{12} & \cdots & \rho_{1k} \\
\rho_{21} & 1 & \cdots & \rho_{2k} \\
\vdots & \vdots & & \vdots \\
\rho_{k1} & \rho_{k2} & \cdots & 1
\end{bmatrix}.
$$

Addition or subtraction of matrices requires that the matrices involved have the same number of rows and the same number of columns. Then the operation is carried out separately on the elements in the ijth position of each matrix, and the result becomes the element of that position in the sum or difference matrix. Multiplication of two matrices $\mathbf{A}$ and $\mathbf{B}$ is possible only if the number of columns in $\mathbf{A}$ is the same as the number of rows in $\mathbf{B}$. Then the matrices are multiplied "rows by columns"; that is, if $\mathbf{A}$ is an $m \times k$ matrix and $\mathbf{B}$ is a $k \times n$ matrix, the product $\mathbf{AB}$ is an $m \times n$ matrix whose ijth element is given by

$$(\mathbf{AB})_{ij} = a_{i1}b_{1i} + \cdots + a_{ik}b_{kj} = \sum_{h=1}^{k} a_{ih}b_{hj}.$$

The multiplication of the $1 \times k$ row vector $[(x_1 - \mu), \ldots, (x_k - \mu)]'$ by its transpose, a $k \times 1$ column vector, yields a 1×1 matrix (called a *scalar*), the sum of squares

$$\sum_{i=1}^{k} (x_i - \mu)^2.$$

However, the multiplication of a $k \times 1$ vector by a $1 \times k$ vector results in a $k \times k$ product matrix. For example, if $\mathbf{a}' = (1,3,4)$ and $\mathbf{b}' = (4,1,2)$, the product

$$\mathbf{ab}' = \begin{bmatrix} 1 \times 4 & 1 \times 1 & 1 \times 2 \\ 3 \times 4 & 3 \times 1 & 3 \times 2 \\ 4 \times 4 & 4 \times 1 & 4 \times 2 \end{bmatrix} = \begin{bmatrix} 4 & 1 & 2 \\ 12 & 3 & 6 \\ 16 & 4 & 8 \end{bmatrix}.$$

Although the operation of division is not defined for matrices, the inverse $\mathbf{A}^{-1}$ of a square matrix $\mathbf{A}$ is defined such that the product $\mathbf{A}^{-1}\mathbf{A} = \mathbf{A}\mathbf{A}^{-1} = \mathbf{I}$, the identity matrix consisting of unities along the main diagonal and zeroes elsewhere. Matrix inversion requires calculation of another quantity also defined only for square matrices called the *determinant* of a matrix and denoted by the absolute number symbol, i.e., $|\mathbf{A}|$ represents the determinant of a square matrix $\mathbf{A}$. Unlike $\mathbf{A}$, which is simply an array of numbers, $|\mathbf{A}|$ is a numerical quantity. Inversion of a $k \times k$ matrix may be executed quickly and accurately by readily available computer programs for any reasonable value of k.

In the bivariate case, the covariance matrix of population parameters, using the familiar notation, is

$$\Sigma = \begin{bmatrix} \sigma_1^2 & \rho_{12}\sigma_1\sigma_2 \\ \rho_{12}\sigma_1\sigma_2 & \sigma_2^2 \end{bmatrix};$$

the inverse of Σ is

$$\Sigma^{-1} = \begin{bmatrix} 1/\sigma_1{}^2(1 - \rho_{12}^2) & -\rho_{12}/\sigma_1\sigma_2(1 - \rho_{12}^2) \\ -\rho_{12}/\sigma_1\sigma_2(1 - \rho_{12}^2) & 1/\sigma_2{}^2(1 - \rho_{12}^2) \end{bmatrix}$$

and the determinant of the inverse is

$$|\Sigma^{-1}| = [\sigma_1{}^2\sigma_2{}^2(1 - \rho_{12}^2)]^{-1}.$$

The reader may verify that the bivariate Normal density function (Equation (4.1)), written in matrix form, becomes

$$f(x_1, x_2) = (1/2\pi)^{-1}|\Sigma^{-1}|^{1/2}\exp\{-\tfrac{1}{2}[(x - \mu)'\Sigma^{-1}(x - \mu)]\},$$

where the vector $(x - \mu)'$ is $[(x_1 - \mu_1), (x_2 - \mu_2)]$.

The probability density function for the multivariate Normal distribution of $k > 2$ variables may similarly be written in the compact matrix notation as

$$f(x) = (1/2\pi)^{-k/2}|\Sigma^{-1}|^{1/2}\exp\{-\tfrac{1}{2}[(x - \mu)'\Sigma^{-1}(x - \mu)]\}, \tag{4.8}$$

where $(x - \mu)'$ and Σ are understood to refer to k variables. Because the random variable in square brackets contains squared as well as linear quantities, it is called a *quadratic form*, denoted here by $\delta_k{}^2$. Transforming x to a vector of independent variables u, as we did in the bivariate case, one may prove that $\delta_k{}^2$ is distributed as chi-square with k degrees of freedom. It follows that setting $\delta_k{}^2$ equal to the $(100p)$th percentile of $\chi_k{}^2$ defines a $100p$ percent MRR for k variables. When $k = 3$, this three-dimensional region is called an ellipsoid; for $k > 3$, the region is called a hyperellipse. When sample estimates must be substituted for the parameters in $\delta_k{}^2$, the region is defined using the F-distribution for k and $(n - k)$ degrees of freedom; that is, the $(100p)$ percent MRR (or better, MPR — multivariate prediction region) includes all k-variate observation vectors contained within the boundary

$$D_k^2 = [k(n^2 - 1)F(p; k, n - k)]/n(n - k), \tag{4.9}$$

where $D_k^2 = (x - \bar{x})'S^{-1}(x - \bar{x})$.

For practical use in the clinical laboratory, we focus on D_k^2. If the general term x is replaced by x_i, representing the k test results for the ith patient, then D_k^2 becomes a multivariate index denoting the "distance" between this patient's profile and the mean profile for the reference population. It is a form of generalized distance, originally developed by Mahalanobis (1936) for discriminating between two populations through a multivariate sample of observations. We then define a multivariate index for interpreting an observed profile vis-à-vis a reference population as

$$D_k^2(x_i) = (x_i - \bar{x})'S^{-1}(x_i - \bar{x}) \tag{4.10}$$

The right-hand side of Equation (4.9) provides a critical value for this index. If $D_k^2(x_i)$ is higher than this value, the patient's multivariate observation lies outside the MPR.

More valuable than a single critical value would be an index that specifies the probability of observing a distance as large or larger than $D_k^2(x_i)$ if the patient were indeed representative of the reference population. Albert (1981) has proposed a quantity that he calls the *atypicality index*, namely,

$$I(x_i) = \text{pr}[D_k^2(x) \leq D_k^2(x_i)]. \tag{4.11}$$

We would suggest instead the complement of this index, say $A(x_i) = 1 - I(x_i)$, because then an unusually large value of $D_k^2(x_i)$ would have a very low probability if the patient were in fact typical of the reference subjects. Analogous to a statistical test of the null hypothesis, a result with a very low probability would indicate a statistically significant finding needing explanation by the laboratory or clinician. Following Albert, $A(x_i)$ may be estimated by the incomplete β-function, $\beta(V_i; k/2; (n - k)/2)$, where $V_i = n/[D^2(x_i) + n]$. As noted in Chapter 2 in connection with the Harrell-Davis percentile estimator, the incomplete β-function is available in statistical programming packages (e.g., the Probbeta procedure in SAS).

In this way, an observed profile of biochemical tests believed to be of diagnostic value can be converted to a single numerical quantity, taking full account of the correlations among the tests. The probability of this result compared to the reference population could be determined through a table lookup function within the laboratory's computing system and listed along with the separate test values (and their reference intervals) on the laboratory report.

We must emphasize that while the greater specificity of the multivariate index compared to multiple univariate reference ranges has potential for reducing the costs of unnecessary follow-up, the index may also "drown out" a warning signal from a single test diagnostic for a particular disease. Diabetes and gout are examples of diseases that present clinically with a single test abnormality (glucose and uric acid, respectively). Boyd and Lacher (1982) showed that as the number of tests included in a multivariate index increases, a larger single-test deviation from the reference mean is required to cause the index to appear abnormal. The required deviation is less when the test of interest is correlated with the remaining tests in the index.

It is important, therefore, that the number of tests included in a multivariate index be fairly small, no more than three or four, that they show significant pairwise correlations, and that they be carefully selected to have good predictive value with respect to a general class of organ-specific diseases (e.g., Sheehan and Haythorn, 1979). It is not likely, for example, that a set of tests showing optimal power to discriminate between two specific liver diseases would be the best set for detecting the presence of any liver disease. In fact, as Solberg et al. (1975) found, the identity of the best biochemical tests for differential diagnosis between liver diseases depends very much on the subset of diseases involved. On the other hand, the differential diagnosis of thyroid disease (e.g., Rootwelt and Solberg, 1981) involves distinguishing between the euthyroid state and either hypo- or hyperthyroidism. In this case, the best discriminating vector of tests is a good candidate for a multivariate index derived from a reference population of euthyroid patients.

4.4 TRANSFORMATION OF VARIABLES

To apply the distance index $D_k^2(\mathbf{x}_i)$, it is not necessary that the variables be jointly distributed in a multivariate Normal distribution. That is, the distance may be computed for each member of the reference sample and the n values ordered by magnitude. Then, population quantiles may be estimated nonparametrically, using, for example, the Harrell-Davis weighted quantile procedure described in Chapter 2. The estimate of the 95th percentile may serve as a reference limit for interpreting the distance index for a new patient.

In addition, the atypicality index A_i may be estimated nonparametrically by interpolating between the p-values associated with estimated percentiles on either side of the patient's distance index and subtracting the interpolated p-value from unity. Durbridge (1983) followed a nonparametric procedure in his experiment described in Section 4.1, but he used the 95 percent sample quantile rather than a more precise estimate as his multivariate reference limit and did not attempt to estimate an atypicality index for each new patient.

An important advantage of the multivariate Normal assumption is that it supports relatively simple yet powerful methods for detecting outlying multivariate vectors. These are less likely to be revealed by visual inspection of the data themselves than are outliers in a univariate distribution. In Section 4.5, we review some of the statistical literature on multivariate outliers.

If we assume that many, perhaps most, biochemical analytes are not Normally distributed across a reference population, finding suitable transformations to produce a joint multivariate Normal distribution for even a small subset of variables is far more difficult than in the univariate case. The problem is that although the marginal density functions of the variables in a multivariate Normal distribution are all univariate Normal, the existence of univariate Normal marginals is not sufficient to assure multivariate Normality.

This means, at least in principle, that we have to determine simultaneously a vector of transformations, for example, by maximizing the likelihood of the (assumed) multivariate Normal distribution after transformation with respect to the transforming parameters. The easier path would be to determine for each variable separately the most suitable transform function to achieve a Normal distribution for that variable. Simultaneous maximum likelihood estimation is not unmanageable in the case of two variables (e.g., Rode and Chinchilli, 1988), but even here, the peak likelihood must be determined in a two-way table of likelihood calculations over a range of transformation parameters for each variable. Johnson and Wichern (1988, Section 4.7) discuss this issue, including an example of the two-variable case, and conclude that maximizing the multivariate Normal likelihood with respect to variation in a vector of transformation parameters is not likely to produce substantially better estimates of these parameters than maximizing the marginal likelihoods.

We suggest that, for practical purposes, the best transformation to a Normal distribution be sought for each variable separately, and the resulting multivariate distance function be tested to see whether it conforms to the chi-square distribution for k degrees of freedom. This assumes that a large number of subjects have been included in the reference sample.

4.5 MULTIVARIATE OUTLIERS

Albert and Harris (1987, Section 2.5) included some discussion of the problem of detecting outliers in a set of multivariate vectors that are otherwise Normally distributed. In particular, they noted two procedures: the graphical method of Healy (1968) and more formal significance tests going back to Wilks (1963). Rather than repeat a general description of these methods, we shall include them in a search for outliers in each of two specific data sets examined in the next section.

A comprehensive review of outlier detection in multivariate data was provided by Gnanadesikan and Kettenring (1972). They pointed out that while univariate outliers simply inflate the estimate of variance, the multivariate variety can affect the distribution in various ways. For example, the values of the individual variables in a multivariate outlier may or may not be atypical, but one pair of variables may exhibit values that do not conform to the covariance or correlation followed by the bulk of other paired observations of those variables.

The detection problem, especially in the case of a small cluster of neighboring outliers, is aggravated by the fact that the sample distance function D_k^2 is not a robust estimator (i.e., resistant to outliers), as was recognized by Gnanadesikan and Kettenring. Thus, a cluster of outliers may attract the multivariate mean in its direction as well as inflate the covariance matrix. The effect of this would be to reduce the estimated distances for the outliers while increasing them for typical observations. In fact, a continuing objective of recent research (e.g., Hadi, 1992, and papers cited therein) has been to obtain more robust distance functions without getting enmeshed in time-consuming, expensive computations. Unfortunately, the methods proposed appear to suffer this burden for sample sizes greater than 100, common in studies undertaken by clinical laboratories.

We mentioned in Chapter 3 (Section 3.4), Healy's (1979) procedure for obtaining a robust estimate of variance by trimming a small proportion of the observations (assuming outliers are present) at both the top and bottom of the distribution. Barnett and Lewis (1994, p. 279) note that robust covariance estimates may be obtained by using the following relationship for any two random variables X_1 and X_2:

$$\text{Cov}(X_1, X_2) = (1/4ab)[\text{Var}(aX_1 + bX_2) - \text{Var}(aX_1 - bX_2)].$$

$$(4.12)$$

Gnanadesikan and Kettenring (1972) suggested $a = [\text{Var}(X_1)]^{-1}$ and $b = [\text{Var}(X_2)]^{-1}$. A robust estimator of $\text{Cov}(X_1, X_2)$ may be obtained by inserting robust estimators of all these variances. These could be obtained through Healy's procedure.

Graphical procedures as part of the process of exploratory examination of the reference data are highly recommended. For example, bivariate scattergrams of pairs of variables (plotting the values of one variable against the corresponding values of another) can help to reveal outliers if the offending variables are strongly correlated in the data set as a whole. Another method, more economical if the number of analytes (k) is at least four or five, is to compute the k principal components (see Appendix 4.1) of the correlation matrix. If at least some of the variables are highly correlated, outliers may show up in bivariate plots of corresponding values of the high-order principal components. On the other hand, if the variables are poorly correlated, such outliers may be revealed in bivariate plots of the low-order components.

We explore applications of some of these methods in the following two examples. They involve a large number of subjects and small multivariate vectors, bivariate and trivariate, typical of what might prove acceptable in clinical practice.

4.6   EXAMPLES

We examine two vectors of analytes: (1) the enzymes alanine transaminase (ALT) and aspartate transaminase (AST), commonly used to measure liver function, and (2) serum creatinine (SCr), urea nitrogen (BUN), and uric acid (UA), indicators of kidney function. Measurements are from single blood specimens obtained from 596 male medical students during the years 1987–1991 at the University of Virginia. The data sets are listed in Appendix 4.1.

The overall correlation between ALT and AST was high (0.75), but this value was inflated by the extreme pair of values seen in the bivariate plot below. The correlations between the renal variables were much lower (SCr-BUN: 0.13; SCr-UA: 0.36; BUN-UA: 0.10), not surprising in these young, physically active subjects. In hunting for outliers, bivariate plots (Figures 4.4 and 4.5) were examined first. Figure 4.4 shows one extremely atypical ALT,AST pair (ALT = 349 U/L, AST = 161 U/L). This subject was later found to be suffering from chronic hepatitis. These observations were deleted from the data set. Figures 4.5a,c indicate an extreme value of BUN (28 mg/dL) accompanied by relatively low creatinine and uric acid. Figures

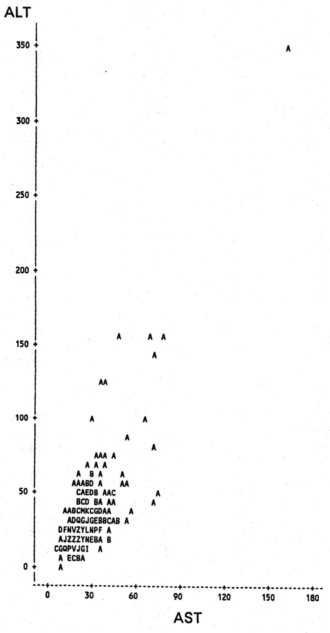

NOTE: 26 observations hidden.

Fig. 4.4 Bivariate plot of liver enzymes: alanine transaminase (ALT) versus aspartate transaminase (AST).

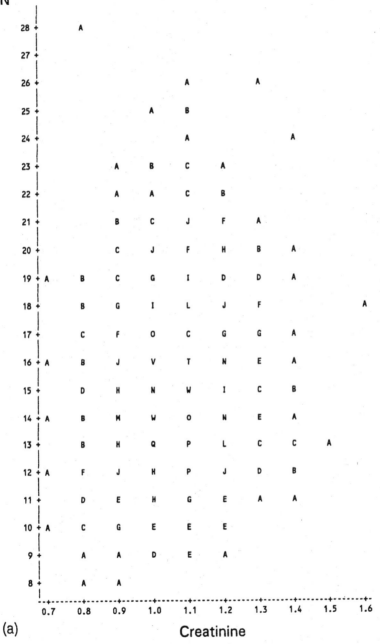

Fig. 4.5 Bivariate plots of renal variables: (a) serum urea nitrogen (BUN) versus serum creatinine (SCr); (b) SCr versus uric acid (UA); (c) BUN versus UA.

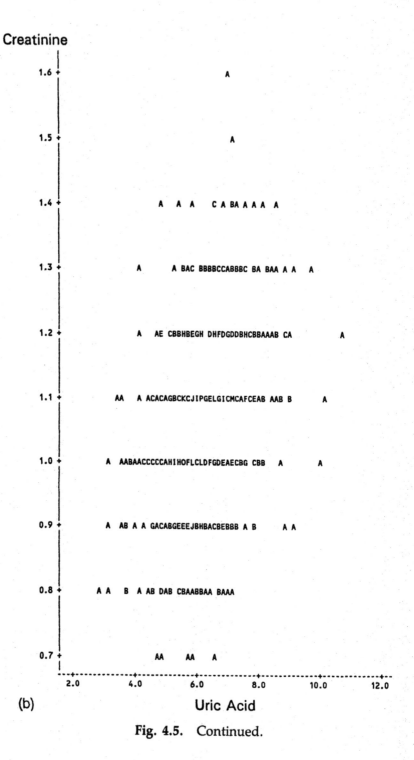

(b)

Fig. 4.5. Continued.

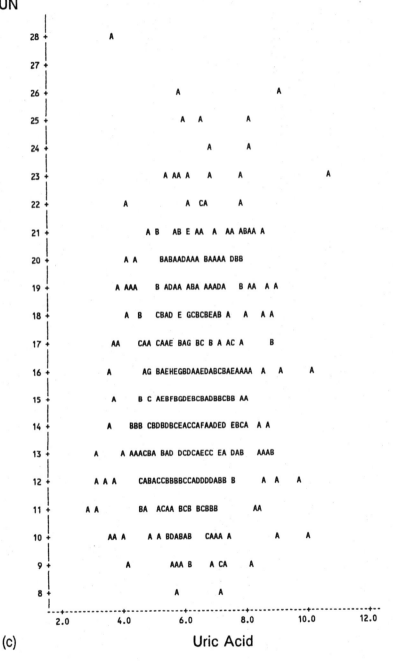

(c)

4.5a,b show an unusually high value of creatinine (1.6 mg/dL), but the corresponding BUN and uric acid concentrations were unremarkable. In Figures 4.5b,c, an unusually high value of uric acid (10.7 mg/dL) appears with a higher than expected BUN (23 mg/dL). None of these renal outliers were deleted at this stage.

4.6.1 Next Steps

Liver Enzymes

The remaining ALT,AST data were transformed into logarithms in an effort to achieve an approximately Normal bivariate distribution as a basis for further testing of outliers. Calculations in Chapter 2 showed the log transform to be appropriate for a smaller sample of ALT data. In the present sample, the log transform reduced the coefficients of skewness in ALT and AST by 92 and 97 percent, respectively, and kurtosis by 89 and 87 percent. Using the logarithms, distance functions $D_2^2(x_i)$ [Equation (4.10)] were computed and their cube roots plotted on Normal probability paper (Figure 4.6). The cube root of a χ^2-distributed variable should be approximately Normally distributed; in this case, the nonlinearity at both ends shows that log ALT, log AST pairs were still not quite distributed in the bivariate Normal form. However, the graph does indicate an additional extreme ALT,AST pair beyond the one already deleted. The observed values were unusually small: ALT = 2, AST = 9 IU/L. The corresponding value of $D_2^2(x_i)$ was 23.5.

Table 4.1 provides 5 percent and 1 percent significance levels of the maximum $D_k^2(x_i)$ for $k = 2$–5 and samples sizes 100(100)500, taken in part from Barnett and Lewis (1994, Table XXXII) and in part from Wilks (1963). Extrapolating to $n = 600$, the estimated 1 percent level was clearly less than the observed value of 23.5. Therefore, this observation vector was also deleted. Recomputing x, S^2, and $D_2^2(x_i)$ for the remaining 594 observations, the maximum $D_2^2(x_i)$ was 15.9, well below the 5 percent level. No further observations were deleted.

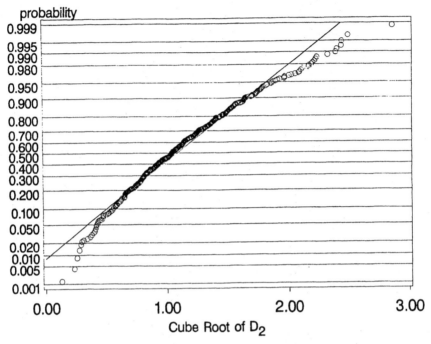

Fig. 4.6 Cumulative distribution of $(D^2)^{1/3}$ for ALT and AST.

Table 4.1 The 5 Percent and 1 Percent Significance Levels for Maximum $D_k^2 (x_i)$ in Testing a Single Outlier from a Multivariate Normal Sample of Size n with $k = 2$ to 5 Variables

	\multicolumn{8}{c}{k}							
	\multicolumn{2}{c}{2}	\multicolumn{2}{c}{3}	\multicolumn{2}{c}{4}	\multicolumn{2}{c}{5}
n	5%	1%	5%	1%	5%	1%	5%	1%
100	14.22	16.95	16.45	19.26	18.43	21.30	20.26	23.17
200	15.99	18.94	18.42	21.47	20.59	23.72	22.59	25.82
300[a]	16.96	19.99	19.48	22.62	21.72	24.96	23.80	27.12
400[a]	17.62	20.69	20.20	23.38	22.48	25.77	24.61	27.98
500	18.12	21.22	20.75	23.95	23.06	26.37	25.21	28.62

[a] Values in this row taken from Wilks (1963) using conversion formulas (7.3.9) and (7.3.10) in Barnett and Lewis (1994, p. 287). Other rows taken from Table XXXII in Barnett and Lewis.

Renal Variables

The renal variables were not transformed because their distributions appeared roughly Normal except for the possible effects of the three outlying observations mentioned earlier. The largest value of D_3^2, 23.05, was associated with the observation vector containing the BUN value of 28 mg/dL. Again extrapolating from Table 4.1, this value appears to approximate the 2 percent level for 600 observations, confirming this observation as a significant outlier.

More interesting is the plot of the first two principal components of the standardized observations (Figure 4.7). The eigenvectors of the correlation matrix associated with these components are, for the first component (0.353_{BUN}, 0.6550_{UA}, 0.6678_{SCr}), and for the second component (0.9334_{BUN}, -0.2934_{UA}, -0.2065_{SCr}). Multiplying these values by the standardized values for the extreme observation (BUN = 28, UA = 3.7, SCr = 0.8), namely, 3.748 for BUN, -2.196 for UA, and -1.843 for SCr) yields the values -1.34 for the first principal component and 4.52 for the second component. This is the outlying point in the northwest corner of Figure 4.7 and represents the unusual association of an extremely high BUN concentration with relatively low UA and SCr concentrations. This observation also shows up as an outlier in the plot of values of the second principal component against the third (Figure 4.8), but the other points are more scattered than in the previous graph, and the contrast is less striking.

This observation was deleted from the set, and the mean vector, covariance matrix and D_3^2 values were recomputed for the remaining observations. The maximum D_3^2, 18.4, was well below the 5 percent significance level. No further observations were deleted.

4.6.2 Summary of Results

Altogether, these procedures recommended three observation vectors for deletion: two liver and one renal. This is a remarka-

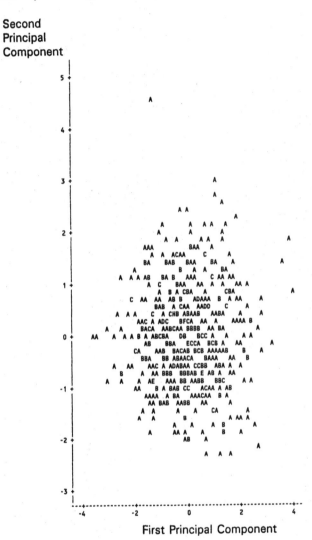

Fig. 4.7 Plot of first two principal components of renal variables.

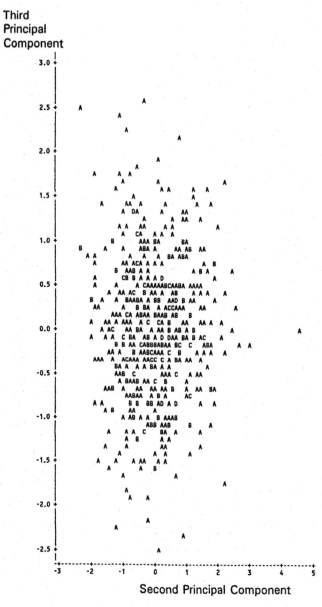

Fig. 4.8 Plot of last two principal components of renal variables.

bly small proportion of the total number, only 0.25 percent. Nevertheless, by substantially decreasing the range of observations, deletion of the two liver vectors lowered the correlation between ALT and AST by 13 percent (from 0.75 to 0.65). Deletion of the extreme BUN value and the rather low values of SCr and UA in the same vector increased the correlation between BUN and SCr by 11 percent (from 0.126 to 0.140) and the correlation between BUN and UA by 16 percent (from 0.098 to 0.114). The correlation between SCr and UA remained at 0.36.

Table 4.2 lists the observed and expected 95th percentiles of D_k^2 after outlier deletion. Expected values were calculated from Equation (4.9).

The multivariate index for the liver enzymes showed a higher than expected 95th percentile, perhaps because the log transforms still retained some skewness and kurtosis. However, recomputing D^2 after applying Box-Cox power transforms (slightly negative, -0.24, for ALT; close to zero, the log transform, for AST) did not change the 95th percentile.

4.6.3 Comparison of BUN/SCr and D_3^2 (Renal)

We noted earlier that the ratio of urea nitrogen to serum creatinine is commonly used by clinicians in differential diagnosis of renal disease and other conditions. Using the present data set, admittedly restricted to young, presumably healthy males, we consider briefly whether the multivariate index including uric acid may provide helpful additional information. First, we examine the statistics of the ratio BUN/SCr. The mean, standard

Table 4.2 Observed and Expected 95th Percentiles of D_k^2

	Liver (D_2^2)	Renal (D_3^2)
Observed	6.84	7.94
Expected	6.04	7.89

deviation, coefficient of variation (CV), and nonparametric (sample quantile) estimates of the 5th and 95th percentiles, based on 595 observations, are listed in Table 4.3. These percentiles agree with the cutpoints of <10 and >20 commonly used by clinicians. The CV agrees closely with that expected from a nonparametric formula for the CV of the ratio R of two variables N and D, namely, $C_R = (C_N^2 + C_D^2 - 2\rho C_N C_D)$. In this case, $C_{BUN} = 21.9\%$, $C_{SCr} = 13.5\%$, and $\rho = 0.14$, yielding an expected C_R of 24.1%.

The mean and standard deviation of the renal multivariate index D_3^2 (BUN, SCr, UA) from these data were 3.0 and 2.54, respectively, compared to expected values of $k = 3$ and $(2k)^{1/2} = 2.45$, where k is the degrees of freedom for the asymptotic chi-square distribution of D_k^2. Figure 4.9 shows the graph of BUN/SCr against D_3^2.

As expected, the vast majority of BUN/SCr ratios between the 5th and 95th percentiles (9.2 and 21) are associated with D^2 values below the 95th percentile, 7.94. The same is true of the majority of BUN/SCr values outside these limits, confirming the conservatism of the multivariate index, although in this case, the comparison is not between the index and the separate variables but between the index and a nonlinear function of two of the variables. Perhaps of greater interest is the finding that observation vectors with D^2 values above the 95th percentile are scattered across the BUN/SCr range, indicating that unusually high multivariate renal indices may offer useful additional diagnostic information, especially with respect to uric acid.

Nine of the thirty high D^2 values correspond to BUN/SCr ratios of ten or below. In four of these nine cases, the UA results

Table 4.3 Statistics of BUN/SCr

Mean	SD	CV (%)	5th percentile	95th percentile
14.5	3.51	24.2	9.2	21

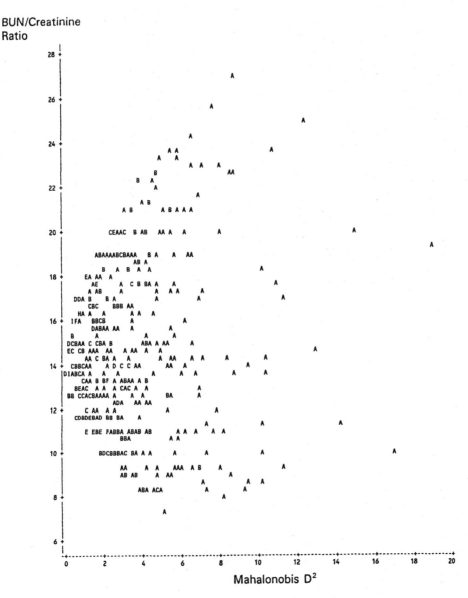

Fig. 4.9 Plot of BUN/SCr ratio versus D^2 index.

were above 8.2 mg/dL, the 95th percentile of UA in these data. The BUN values were low (10–13 mg/dL); SCr values were average to high (1.0–1.4 mg/dL). In eight of the high D^2 occurrences, the BUN/SCr ratio equaled or exceeded 20. The highest UA values in this group were 8.2 and 9.1 mg/dL, associated with high BUN values: 25 and 26 mg/dL, respectively.

The remaining 13 instances of high D^2 values with BUN/SCr values greater than 10 or less than 20, essentially within the 90 percent reference range for the ratio, were often characterized by unusually high or unusually low UA values. In five cases, the UA result was in the range 8.2–10.7 mg/dL; in one of these, both BUN and SCr were also high (24 and 1.4 mg/dL). In five other cases, the UA value was below 4.4 mg/dL, the 5th percentile; in two of these, BUN and SCr were also low (11 and 0.8 mg/dL in both cases). Of the three remaining vectors, two showed unusually high values of SCr (1.4 and 1.6 mg/dL) although not quite high enough to bring the BUN/SCr ratio to 10 or below, and one included an unusually low combination of BUN and SCr values (10 and 0.7 mg/dl).

In sum, these results confirm the high specificity of the multivariate index, but also imply, as Durbridge found from his study, that reporting values of D^2 exceeding the 95th percentile may usefully alert some clinicians to reconsider laboratory test results that might otherwise have been passed over.

APPENDIX 4.1 EIGENVALUES, EIGENVECTORS, AND PRINCIPAL COMPONENTS

The eigenvalues of a $k \times k$ square matrix $\mathbf{A}$ are the solutions $\lambda_1, \lambda_2, \ldots, \lambda_k$ of the determinantal equation $|\mathbf{A} - \lambda \mathbf{I}| = 0$, where $\mathbf{I}$ is the $k \times k$ identity matrix. For the bivariate correlation matrix

$$\boldsymbol{\rho}_2 = \begin{bmatrix} 1 & \rho_{12} \\ \rho_{21} & 1 \end{bmatrix}, \quad (\rho_{12} = \rho_{21})$$

$$\boldsymbol{\rho}_2 - \lambda \mathbf{I} = \begin{bmatrix} 1 - \lambda & \rho_{12} \\ \rho_{21} & 1 - \lambda \end{bmatrix}$$

and the determinantal equation $|\boldsymbol{\rho}_2 - \lambda \mathbf{I}| = (1 - \lambda)^2 - \rho_{12}^2 = 0$ has the solutions (or roots) $\lambda_1 = 1 + \rho_{12}$, $\lambda_2 = 1 - \rho_{12}$. The sum of the eigenvalues equals the number of variables.

Let λ be an eigenvalue of the $k \times k$ matrix $\mathbf{A}$. Now, if $\boldsymbol{\epsilon}$ is a nonzero $k \times 1$ vector (i.e., at least one element of $\boldsymbol{\epsilon}$ is nonzero) satisfying the equation $\mathbf{A}\boldsymbol{\epsilon} = \lambda \boldsymbol{\epsilon}$, then $\boldsymbol{\epsilon}$ is called an eigenvector of $\mathbf{A}$ associated with the eigenvalue λ. In the bivariate case, where $\mathbf{A}$ is taken to be $\boldsymbol{\rho}_2$, the eigenvector $\boldsymbol{\epsilon}_1' = (e_{11}, e_{12})$ associated with the eigenvalue $\lambda_1 = 1 + \rho_{12}$ is given by

$$\begin{bmatrix} 1 & \rho_{12} \\ \rho_{21} & 1 \end{bmatrix} \begin{bmatrix} e_{11} \\ e_{12} \end{bmatrix} = (1 + \rho_{12}) \begin{bmatrix} e_{11} \\ e_{12} \end{bmatrix},$$

or $e_{11} = e_{12}$. Since the elements of an eigenvector are usually "normalized," so that their squares sum to unity, $\boldsymbol{\epsilon}_1' = (1/\sqrt{2}, 1/\sqrt{2})$. Similarly, the eigenvector $\boldsymbol{\epsilon}_2' = (e_{21}, e_{22})$ associated with the eigenvalue $\lambda_2 = 1 - \rho_{12}$ is given by $\boldsymbol{\epsilon}_2' = (1/\sqrt{2}, -1/\sqrt{2})$.

The principal components of a set of observation vectors of k variables are the equations of the axes of the k-dimensional surfaces of constant probability (e.g., in the bivariate Normal case, the major and minor axes of the ellipses illustrated in Figure 4.3). If the original variables are correlated with each other, as would be true in general, then the k principal components are linear transforms of these variables to new variables that are uncorrelated with each other. When the original variables are in standardized form $\mathbf{z}' = (z_1, z_2, \ldots, z_k)$, the principal components, say, $y_1, y_2, \ldots, y_k$, are obtained from the eigenvectors of the correlation matrix $\boldsymbol{\rho}_k$, according to the formula, $y_i = \boldsymbol{\epsilon}_i' \mathbf{z}$. In the bivariate case,

$$y_1 = (1/\sqrt{2}, 1/\sqrt{2})(z_1, z_2)' = (z_1/\sqrt{2}) + (z_2/\sqrt{2}),$$

$$y_2 = (z_1/\sqrt{2}) - (z_2/\sqrt{2}).$$

The variance of the component y_i is equal to the eigenvalue λ_i. Therefore, if one wants to transform the original standardized variables to a set of uncorrelated variables with unit variance, say, $u_1, u_2, \ldots, u_k$, as was desired in Section 4.2, then the formulas $u_i = (1/\lambda_i)^{1/2}\epsilon_i'z$ should be used, leading, in the bivariate case, to Equations (4.4).

APPENDIX 4.2   DATA ON LIVER ENZYMES: ALANINE TRANSAMINASE AND ASPARTATE TRANSAMINASE (ALT, AST) AND RENAL VARIABLES: UREA NITROGEN, SERUM CREATININE, URIC ACID (BUN, SCr, UA)

Data begins on p. 137.

OBS	ALT	AST	BUN	SCR	UA
1	21	19	26	1.1	5.9
2	31	34	18	1.0	7.1
3	34	30	13	1.2	6.5
4	16	21	15	1.3	7.4
5	23	25	21	1.1	6.2
6	26	15	13	1.1	7.5
7	24	23	14	1.1	6.0
8	18	14	18	1.1	6.8
9	51	27	17	1.1	6.0
10	103	31	15	1.1	7.5
11	23	9	12	1.1	5.4
12	28	21	13	1.2	8.9
13	124	39	15	1.0	5.9
14	30	21	18	1.3	6.3
15	34	26	20	1.2	7.3
16	123	37	16	1.0	5.6
17	26	23	12	1.2	7.5
18	24	32	14	1.0	4.4
19	16	30	17	1.3	7.8
20	35	41	20	1.2	7.8
21	15	35	16	1.2	6.0
22	102	66	18	1.3	8.9
23	90	53	15	1.2	7.0
24	62	52	17	1.0	5.6
25	21	28	12	0.9	6.2
26	29	35	14	1.0	7.6
27	13	20	16	1.2	7.6
28	19	32	15	1.3	5.7
29	55	55	10	0.9	5.7
30	19	37	9	1.1	8.2
31	23	35	22	1.2	6.7
32	19	30	21	1.1	6.5
33	66	39	9	1.1	6.9
34	28	29	20	1.2	6.0
35	45	26	14	1.2	7.3
36	24	32	14	1.0	4.4
37	30	38	14	1.1	6.3
38	30	29	11	1.0	5.3
39	25	27	13	1.2	6.0
40	22	20	11	0.9	7.0
41	29	27	12	1.1	7.1
42	4	16	12	1.1	5.1
43	33	26	24	1.4	8.2
44	155	47	16	1.3	5.5
45	35	32	16	1.2	5.1
46	25	28	14	1.1	7.0
47	27	32	13	1.1	6.1
48	42	24	15	1.2	7.3
49	30	23	20	1.0	6.4
50	42	34	16	1.2	8.6

OBS	ALT	AST	BUN	SCR	UA
51	14	25	16	1.0	4.9
52	24	18	14	1.2	6.1
53	21	14	17	1.0	6.1
54	31	27	14	1.1	8.4
55	10	12	13	1.1	6.1
56	50	46	13	1.3	7.6
57	24	9	14	1.0	5.0
58	19	23	10	1.2	7.4
59	32	21	14	1.3	7.3
60	21	17	17	0.9	5.3
61	20	23	14	1.2	7.5
62	349	161	10	1.0	10.0
63	20	25	15	1.1	5.5
64	33	19	15	1.1	6.2
65	13	10	10	1.1	5.6
66	22	19	15	1.2	4.9
67	22	11	10	0.9	6.2
68	14	12	16	1.1	8.2
69	20	17	13	1.2	4.9
70	22	12	14	1.3	7.3
71	18	21	14	1.4	5.8
72	13	19	17	1.1	5.1
73	22	20	22	1.2	4.2
74	37	28	18	1.2	8.5
75	20	23	18	0.9	5.4
76	34	21	16	1.0	6.6
77	18	13	18	1.2	6.1
78	32	29	12	1.2	6.4
79	17	22	17	1.2	5.5
80	35	26	16	1.0	7.4
81	20	11	18	1.2	6.8
82	32	27	17	1.0	5.9
83	23	8	23	1.0	7.8
84	40	27	17	0.9	6.8
85	14	13	11	1.2	4.7
86	24	16	12	1.1	6.5
87	20	21	15	1.1	7.2
88	21	15	13	1.0	5.8
89	20	17	13	1.2	6.0
90	27	21	13	0.9	3.2
91	28	22	22	1.1	6.5
92	24	18	21	0.9	4.9
93	23	16	14	1.0	7.9
94	51	26	14	0.9	5.9
95	39	20	12	1.0	5.7
96	75	39	9	1.1	7.2
97	25	12	19	1.2	7.1
98	18	19	9	1.0	5.7
99	34	27	12	1.1	6.9
100	40	13	15	1.1	6.0

OBS	ALT	AST	BUN	SCR	UA
101	20	11	13	1.0	7.1
102	25	27	18	1.2	5.6
103	24	32	19	1.3	7.9
104	37	57	13	1.0	6.3
105	16	22	18	1.2	6.7
106	6	24	18	1.3	8.0
107	51	27	19	1.0	6.1
108	25	41	12	0.8	3.7
109	39	36	21	1.2	6.1
110	23	17	12	1.4	5.4
111	19	20	18	0.9	6.3
112	23	18	10	0.9	3.7
113	37	27	8	0.8	7.2
114	28	30	16	1.1	10.2
115	19	16	13	1.2	7.6
116	22	21	17	0.9	3.7
117	30	29	13	1.3	6.5
118	15	13	12	1.2	7.6
119	36	28	16	1.2	6.6
120	49	74	12	1.3	8.6
121	69	34	11	1.1	6.4
122	15	18	15	1.1	6.9
123	16	18	18	0.9	6.5
124	37	30	15	1.1	5.9
125	18	21	13	1.0	5.5
126	54	36	17	0.9	6.9
127	36	24	17	1.2	8.9
128	25	17	18	1.1	6.1
129	18	21	17	1.3	6.4
130	25	26	20	0.9	5.8
131	19	16	20	1.2	6.0
132	22	20	16	1.0	5.6
133	39	35	19	0.8	6.3
134	53	30	15	1.0	6.4
135	24	19	11	0.8	3.2
136	24	17	25	1.0	8.2
137	31	41	25	1.1	6.6
138	55	28	21	1.0	8.0
139	25	28	16	1.0	7.5
140	31	41	12	0.9	6.0
141	35	25	13	1.2	5.3
142	19	17	12	1.2	6.7
143	36	32	12	0.9	6.1
144	33	20	18	0.8	5.1
145	84	72	18	1.0	6.4
146	18	20	11	1.1	6.7
147	14	16	13	1.0	4.7
148	24	24	19	1.2	8.1
149	36	28	11	1.2	8.3
150	21	24	21	1.1	5.7

OBS	ALT	AST	BUN	SCR	UA
151	20	41	26	1.3	9.1
152	31	34	22	1.0	6.5
153	13	26	12	1.3	9.7
154	14	22	17	1.0	4.6
155	12	20	14	1.2	5.4
156	17	26	13	1.1	7.2
157	16	19	16	1.0	7.3
158	22	19	19	1.1	8.7
159	35	24	13	0.8	4.4
160	26	32	14	1.0	7.5
161	31	21	17	0.9	4.6
162	16	23	16	1.1	6.0
163	27	32	21	1.2	5.8
164	78	33	20	1.2	7.6
165	33	27	13	1.1	7.3
166	21	28	16	1.1	6.2
167	42	33	14	1.0	8.0
168	49	42	14	1.1	7.6
169	33	27	18	0.9	5.5
170	16	22	21	1.2	8.0
171	14	26	12	1.2	5.3
172	20	22	25	1.1	6.0
173	20	23	11	1.2	6.4
174	36	36	10	1.2	7.0
175	22	32	14	1.2	6.2
176	36	23	14	1.1	8.7
177	159	77	11	1.1	6.0
178	36	33	12	0.9	4.6
179	48	31	13	1.0	6.8
180	60	36	14	1.0	5.7
181	28	23	14	1.0	5.2
182	16	25	18	1.2	6.6
183	22	31	13	1.2	6.7
184	24	36	16	1.1	7.2
185	35	28	15	1.1	7.0
186	22	25	12	1.3	5.9
187	25	30	20	1.0	4.4
188	35	25	18	1.1	6.5
189	31	30	13	1.1	4.7
190	16	24	17	1.2	6.1
191	29	42	19	1.1	7.3
192	19	13	16	1.1	5.5
193	27	35	19	1.2	7.0
194	20	32	15	0.9	5.9
195	39	34	20	1.0	5.3
196	25	32	17	1.3	5.9
197	37	35	21	1.0	8.1
198	23	29	18	1.1	7.2
199	33	46	11	1.0	6.0
200	30	53	13	1.1	6.9

OBS	ALT	AST	BUN	SCR	UA
201	47	29	18	1.1	6.3
202	17	18	14	1.0	4.3
203	20	23	16	1.4	4.8
204	26	26	12	1.1	3.4
205	30	29	19	1.1	7.8
206	19	26	22	1.1	7.8
207	31	20	21	1.1	8.5
208	14	20	12	1.1	6.5
209	20	18	23	1.0	5.4
210	11	9	16	1.2	6.9
211	26	24	15	1.2	8.0
212	36	21	16	1.1	7.0
213	14	16	14	1.1	6.3
214	24	14	14	0.9	6.5
215	31	20	16	1.2	4.8
216	54	19	15	1.1	7.8
217	25	23	19	1.1	4.4
218	27	24	16	1.0	4.8
219	33	25	18	1.1	5.9
220	19	16	13	1.1	5.4
221	19	17	18	1.3	5.3
222	20	20	18	1.3	6.9
223	10	21	19	1.3	8.3
224	16	29	13	1.4	8.5
225	21	17	15	1.0	5.4
226	11	23	12	1.2	7.3
227	30	24	15	1.0	5.2
228	20	15	12	1.1	5.0
229	18	23	13	1.4	7.9
230	12	20	12	1.1	4.9
231	13	10	11	1.2	6.0
232	13	27	15	0.9	5.3
233	21	22	15	1.1	5.3
234	39	24	14	1.0	7.6
235	8	16	20	1.2	7.0
236	15	23	16	1.1	6.7
237	18	16	23	1.1	5.8
238	35	25	21	1.3	8.3
239	17	10	16	1.3	5.8
240	19	28	18	1.3	4.2
241	9	8	19	1.3	6.4
242	21	15	15	1.4	7.3
243	18	20	20	1.2	6.7
244	10	7	16	1.3	7.2
245	10	15	18	1.0	5.8
246	15	13	17	1.3	6.1
247	45	23	12	1.2	6.6
248	25	23	18	1.1	4.6
249	19	14	12	1.2	5.2
250	20	12	14	1.1	5.2

OBS	ALT	AST	BUN	SCR	UA
251	15	9	14	1.2	7.7
252	41	27	11	1.1	5.5
253	27	16	9	1.2	6.1
254	36	14	19	1.2	6.7
255	20	25	15	1.1	6.3
256	24	18	13	1.0	6.7
257	15	11	13	1.1	7.5
258	11	12	17	1.1	6.1
259	27	18	15	1.0	7.3
260	21	27	20	1.1	7.7
261	21	14	19	0.9	4.3
262	11	11	15	1.1	6.8
263	17	20	13	1.4	6.6
264	16	16	16	1.3	6.5
265	18	13	15	1.0	3.7
266	26	25	15	1.2	5.6
267	73	37	19	1.1	9.0
268	15	9	17	1.0	6.5
269	38	20	16	1.1	7.3
270	15	11	21	1.1	7.4
271	22	9	16	1.0	5.4
272	11	7	15	0.9	6.2
273	13	17	17	1.0	4.7
274	9	17	13	1.1	6.6
275	10	13	11	1.4	6.6
276	19	20	17	1.2	8.8
277	19	23	17	1.2	7.5
278	13	24	10	1.2	6.0
279	33	21	20	1.1	7.9
280	25	20	11	0.8	5.4
281	55	31	16	1.0	6.1
282	48	31	14	1.2	6.5
283	158	68	16	1.1	7.6
284	27	14	19	1.1	6.3
285	13	19	14	1.0	5.4
286	18	16	13	1.2	7.7
287	14	15	15	1.1	6.0
288	12	22	12	1.1	9.0
289	19	19	12	1.2	7.0
290	34	40	21	1.1	5.2
291	40	30	17	1.3	6.1
292	11	14	14	0.9	4.9
293	15	12	21	1.1	6.2
294	19	15	16	1.1	7.7
295	12	12	14	1.2	5.4
296	31	22	13	1.2	6.9
297	17	13	14	1.0	3.6
298	28	17	15	1.1	6.6
299	15	12	13	1.2	6.5
300	38	19	15	1.1	6.7

OBS	ALT	AST	BUN	SCR	UA
301	47	26	13	1.3	8.4
302	14	10	15	1.2	5.5
303	19	18	16	1.2	6.2
304	22	20	14	1.0	5.3
305	17	17	18	1.2	5.9
306	26	19	16	1.2	5.7
307	14	15	12	1.1	6.4
308	60	22	12	1.1	4.5
309	49	40	15	1.0	5.3
310	21	25	15	1.1	4.6
311	19	20	15	1.2	6.9
312	57	23	15	1.1	5.6
313	20	21	23	1.2	10.7
314	15	26	12	1.1	6.4
315	36	18	21	0.9	5.9
316	19	27	14	1.1	4.8
317	27	30	20	1.3	5.6
318	23	19	19	1.4	7.2
319	19	17	11	1.3	6.9
320	27	35	17	1.3	7.4
321	37	38	16	1.1	5.5
322	15	19	18	1.2	6.1
323	21	17	15	1.1	6.1
324	11	7	13	1.1	5.9
325	23	19	14	1.3	6.3
326	20	16	11	1.1	6.6
327	56	30	13	1.1	7.1
328	21	16	10	1.1	3.6
329	28	23	17	1.0	6.2
330	23	18	17	1.0	3.9
331	14	15	18	1.1	5.2
332	16	20	13	1.1	6.7
333	26	32	19	1.1	5.6
334	20	14	13	1.1	5.6
335	25	31	10	1.0	5.4
336	25	22	14	1.1	5.6
337	20	17	14	1.0	6.1
338	32	15	15	1.1	7.2
339	18	26	14	1.2	7.2
340	21	20	11	1.1	6.6
341	22	14	22	1.1	6.1
342	27	29	11	1.2	8.4
343	23	22	19	1.0	5.6
344	30	23	9	1.1	7.2
345	13	11	16	1.0	5.6
346	20	27	10	1.1	5.5
347	141	73	10	0.9	6.7
348	44	27	12	1.0	6.3
349	55	26	15	1.4	6.5
350	36	23	17	1.2	5.6

OBS	ALT	AST	BUN	SCR	UA
351	14	17	14	1.0	4.3
352	19	20	20	1.4	7.5
353	22	22	16	1.2	7.9
354	18	19	20	1.1	6.3
355	17	18	12	1.1	5.7
356	34	30	12	1.4	6.9
357	19	25	15	1.3	6.8
358	42	21	19	1.3	7.2
359	61	30	15	1.1	6.0
360	23	12	13	1.1	6.3
361	22	19	16	1.3	6.7
362	12	15	12	1.3	6.7
363	24	14	14	1.2	7.1
364	18	16	16	1.2	5.5
365	26	21	18	1.6	7.0
366	14	17	16	1.2	4.9
367	48	45	10	1.1	7.1
368	17	23	14	1.2	6.6
369	19	15	16	1.2	5.2
370	27	23	13	1.0	8.7
371	14	27	12	1.2	5.5
372	8	22	17	1.4	7.1
373	28	14	10	1.1	6.7
374	23	11	11	1.0	5.2
375	22	12	14	1.1	5.8
376	16	11	15	1.0	6.3
377	23	15	12	1.0	3.2
378	22	15	16	1.1	6.5
379	31	20	23	1.1	6.8
380	17	19	10	1.2	5.5
381	23	33	10	1.2	9.0
382	53	32	20	1.2	7.1
383	20	20	14	1.3	7.0
384	23	31	15	1.1	6.4
385	21	22	15	1.1	6.1
386	12	19	17	1.3	7.5
387	44	21	11	1.0	5.3
388	12	14	18	1.2	5.9
389	31	24	14	1.2	6.4
390	21	24	19	1.0	3.8
391	27	21	12	1.0	6.0
392	26	20	13	1.0	4.0
393	17	18	13	1.0	5.6
394	17	19	16	1.1	4.8
395	20	23	24	1.1	6.9
396	48	22	14	0.9	5.5
397	17	15	18	0.8	5.1
398	16	19	18	1.1	6.7
399	20	17	12	0.9	7.3
400	16	16	15	1.0	5.6

OBS	ALT	AST	BUN	SCR	UA
401	18	28	13	0.9	7.1
402	27	29	16	1.1	8.0
403	20	17	13	1.0	5.3
404	29	20	14	1.0	7.0
405	22	17	13	0.9	8.9
406	12	18	15	1.0	5.6
407	18	19	11	0.9	6.1
408	14	18	15	0.9	6.1
409	29	22	12	1.1	5.3
410	13	12	14	0.9	4.8
411	26	19	16	0.9	3.6
412	26	19	16	1.1	5.8
413	17	20	20	1.1	5.5
414	18	21	12	1.0	6.7
415	19	24	9	1.0	7.1
416	33	33	17	1.2	6.5
417	25	31	12	1.0	7.1
418	37	26	18	0.9	5.6
419	33	19	19	1.1	5.8
420	14	20	11	0.9	4.5
421	24	32	21	1.2	7.0
422	23	23	20	1.0	5.7
423	24	23	12	0.8	6.1
424	13	14	15	1.0	5.9
425	17	22	16	1.1	7.5
426	27	20	9	1.0	7.3
427	15	16	23	0.9	5.7
428	23	28	19	1.1	4.2
429	22	21	15	0.9	5.3
430	20	23	14	1.0	6.5
431	39	25	10	1.0	5.6
432	16	20	16	0.9	5.4
433	28	22	14	0.9	7.0
434	20	15	16	1.0	6.5
435	20	18	16	1.0	6.4
436	25	24	16	0.9	6.2
437	37	27	15	1.2	7.4
438	19	13	15	0.9	5.7
439	11	19	13	1.0	6.3
440	20	21	12	0.7	4.9
441	22	15	14	0.9	5.0
442	27	22	13	1.0	4.3
443	16	18	16	0.8	5.4
444	28	28	18	1.0	5.6
445	15	14	18	1.2	5.8
446	20	17	17	0.8	6.2
447	21	20	21	1.0	6.2
448	47	33	9	0.9	5.8
449	19	15	15	0.8	4.6
450	23	20	10	0.8	6.8

OBS	ALT	AST	BUN	SCR	UA
451	20	17	9	1.1	6.1
452	25	21	17	1.0	6.5
453	13	11	12	1.0	4.7
454	16	28	13	0.9	7.9
455	16	18	14	1.0	5.2
456	31	18	19	1.0	5.2
457	21	25	9	1.0	5.5
458	14	16	11	1.0	4.6
459	17	17	17	1.0	5.6
460	22	21	14	0.8	4.6
461	15	14	10	0.8	4.9
462	29	22	14	1.0	6.6
463	26	27	21	1.1	6.1
464	13	19	20	1.1	6.7
465	7	17	14	1.0	7.9
466	12	15	14	0.9	5.4
467	68	28	13	1.1	6.0
468	40	27	10	0.7	5.8
469	40	32	16	1.1	5.7
470	31	19	16	1.1	5.4
471	15	15	12	0.9	5.8
472	36	25	16	0.9	6.3
473	17	19	14	0.9	5.3
474	20	19	20	1.0	4.1
475	37	26	23	1.1	6.2
476	58	52	14	1.3	6.7
477	12	18	9	0.8	4.2
478	18	15	15	1.0	5.4
479	11	19	21	1.1	5.2
480	26	33	20	1.0	5.3
481	26	20	17	1.0	6.4
482	22	19	17	1.0	5.2
483	20	22	13	1.0	5.9
484	31	28	12	0.9	4.6
485	17	19	15	0.8	4.8
486	25	24	16	1.0	4.9
487	25	21	18	0.9	6.8
488	42	45	10	0.9	4.0
489	15	19	12	0.8	6.7
490	29	20	19	0.9	5.2
491	25	15	10	0.9	5.4
492	35	25	13	0.8	5.0
493	15	18	10	0.9	6.7
494	30	27	21	1.1	7.9
495	28	31	18	1.0	7.4
496	21	30	16	0.7	4.7
497	44	73	28	0.8	3.7
498	54	30	14	1.0	5.9
499	42	36	16	0.9	9.1
500	23	24	17	0.8	5.6

OBS	ALT	AST	BUN	SCR	UA
501	10	19	19	1.0	6.9
502	37	29	20	1.3	7.5
503	14	18	13	1.0	6.1
504	23	29	17	1.0	5.2
505	18	29	14	0.9	5.8
506	22	22	20	1.0	5.4
507	16	20	16	1.0	5.7
508	61	30	8	0.9	5.7
509	10	9	16	0.9	5.3
510	44	27	10	1.0	5.1
511	16	25	12	1.1	6.5
512	40	25	15	0.9	5.9
513	17	17	16	0.9	7.6
514	28	32	15	1.1	6.4
515	18	17	20	1.0	6.0
516	32	22	14	0.8	5.7
517	7	17	13	1.0	6.2
518	11	28	17	0.9	4.5
519	35	24	20	1.0	6.2
520	48	28	18	1.0	5.3
521	50	23	12	1.0	6.8
522	29	48	16	0.9	5.7
523	30	32	19	0.8	5.4
524	38	33	14	1.1	7.1
525	17	13	15	0.8	4.8
526	17	15	12	0.9	5.3
527	27	24	15	1.0	5.9
528	14	28	11	0.9	6.2
529	20	21	16	1.0	5.8
530	18	27	10	0.8	5.8
531	24	34	12	0.9	6.9
532	33	20	12	0.8	6.4
533	18	18	11	0.8	2.8
534	16	20	14	1.1	7.2
535	45	25	14	0.9	7.3
536	28	14	16	1.0	5.6
537	16	24	16	1.2	7.0
538	12	17	17	1.0	5.4
539	27	23	18	1.0	6.4
540	23	31	15	1.2	5.9
541	18	22	16	1.0	5.9
542	43	41	14	0.7	6.5
543	30	25	13	1.0	4.5
544	19	28.	16	0.9	7.1
545	36	33	15	1.0	7.6
546	21	43	13	1.5	7.2
547	26	26	11	1.1	5.8
548	7	16	16	1.1	5.9
549	26	25	18	1.1	6.8
550	2	9	14	1.1	5.1

OBS	ALT	AST	BUN	SCR	UA
551	13	18	14	1.0	6.8
552	11	18	10	1.0	6.1
553	20	23	11	1.0	6.7
554	26	22	11	1.0	5.3
555	72	45	20	1.0	7.6
556	6	16	18	1.0	6.1
557	8	21	16	0.9	5.4
558	6	15	13	0.9	5.5
559	10	22	21	1.2	7.5
560	30	23	11	1.0	6.9
561	47	21	17	0.8	4.9
562	19	24	16	0.8	6.7
563	32	47	16	1.0	5.7
564	12	25	11	0.8	7.0
565	14	23	20	1.1	7.7
566	33	33	19	0.9	5.6
567	24	36	14	1.1	7.2
568	12	25	12	0.8	6.0
569	12	22	13	1.2	4.8
570	21	19	13	0.9	4.7
571	22	22	15	0.9	5.3
572	12	13	19	1.0	7.2
573	28	33	19	0.7	5.7
574	55	31	22	0.9	6.6
575	13	27	18	0.9	4.6
576	16	15	20	0.9	6.0
577	25	32	20	0.9	6.8
578	14	19	16	1.0	5.9
579	26	24	18	1.1	6.2
580	55	22	18	1.0	6.1
581	28	25	19	1.0	5.6
582	14	27	18	1.1	6.1
583	23	26	14	0.9	4.6
584	21	26	12	0.9	5.2
585	25	23	13	0.9	5.8
586	24	24	12	0.8	5.5
587	52	21	15	0.8	6.0
588	53	44	16	1.0	5.8
589	28	35	14	1.2	7.7
590	25	26	14	0.9	7.9
591	34	22	14	1.2	5.7
592	20	18	11	0.9	5.9
593	18	19	17	1.0	7.5
594	16	18	16	1.0	6.7
595	33	37	21	1.2	6.4
596	23	19	13	0.9	6.4

5

TIME-DEPENDENT REFERENCE VALUES

5.1 INTRODUCTION

In Chapter 3, Section 3.3, we proposed some statistical criteria to assess the need for reference ranges of a biochemical analyte in subgroups of the population, (e.g., by age or gender). The general theme was that group-specific ranges had to justify themselves first on clinical or physiological grounds and then by passing statistical significance tests more stringent than those usually applied to test differences between group means.

In some other areas of human biology, such as physical anthropology or the educational attainments of children, it is taken for granted that measurements change with age and are often dependent on gender and environment. Familiar examples are the charts of "standard" height and weight percentiles for each year of age in boys and girls or each month in neonates.

Changes in selected biochemistries during infancy and childhood have also been recognized and analyzed, for example, in serum creatinine (Savory, 1990), immunoglobulins (Irjala et al., 1990), and amylase isoenzymes (Gillard et al., 1983). In these investigations, the data for different age groups were obtained through cross-sectional studies, each subject providing a single sample for biochemical analysis. A longitudinal study, on the other hand, is characterized by repeated measurements of each subject over time. For example, O'Leary et al. (1991) measured changes in reproductive hormones during normal pregnancy, collecting three blood samples from each woman, one during each trimester of pregnancy. An earlier report by Winkel et al. (1976) analyzed plasma progesterone concentrations in a very small number of women sampled frequently during their pregnancies. They also computed time-dependent reference percentiles based on cross-sectional (single-sample) results from several hundred women at different times during pregnancy.

In cross-sectional studies of an age-dependent variable, the primary objective is to estimate selected percentiles of the distribution of values at any given age or within narrow age bands. Healy (1988) noted that anthropometric measurements of linear distances, such as height or limb length are often approximately Normally distributed at any age. Therefore, the custom in this field has been to obtain means and standard deviations within each age group, smooth these statistics by eye or by curve fitting, and then calculate Normal estimators of desired percentiles at each age. For variables like weight or girth, where distributions are generally not Normal, nonparametric quantile estimators may be computed, as described in Chapter 2. However, unless large numbers of subjects at the same age have been measured, such estimators as $Q_{0.025}$ and $Q_{0.975}$ will be strongly influenced by extreme observations.

When percentile estimates have been obtained separately for each age group, they may be joined by straight lines, producing continuous, if disjointed, charts to aid in interpreting a measurement in a new subject. A unique collection of such charts for biochemical analytes is the *Atlas of Blood Data* prepared by Munan et al. (1978) based on a randomly selected sample of 900 households (totaling 2378 persons) in an area of Quebec during 1974. Fourteen common serum analytes and three hematological variables were measured in each subject. Quantile estimates of 5th, 20th, 50th, 80th, and 95th percentiles were charted for each analyte by 4-year age groups and each sex from 10 to 14 years through 75 years and over.

This was a pioneering study, but, as the previously cited references indicate, there is a growing interest among clinical chemists and clinicians for more detailed percentile information on the distribution of various analytes among healthy persons in narrow age groups, especially during early years or special physiological circumstances such as pregnancy or menopause. Indeed, it is well recognized that many analytes show continuous, sometimes complicated, changes throughout a healthy lifetime, as evidenced in recent texts on pediatric reference values and on reference values in the elderly (Meites, 1989; Faulkner and Meites, 1994).

During the past decade, statisticians and others analyzing measurements of growth and other dynamic processes have published a variety of new methods for estimating and smoothing centile[1] curves as functions of age. Most have been applied to physical measurements, but should also be considered for biochemical data. These methods, like those discussed in Chapter 2, may be classed as parametric or nonparametric. The distinction here is rather fuzzy, however. Although the nonparametric methods make no assumption about the mathematical form of the distribution at a given age, they do involve smoothing the estimated centiles, and the smoothing functions include parameters to be estimated (e.g., the coefficients of a polynomial). Such procedures are sometimes called quasi-parametric, but we will continue the nonparametric designation. The parametric methods attempt to Normalize the distribution of the variable within each age bracket or over the entire age span. Then, Normal estimators are used to derive the centile curves.

In Sections 5.2 and 5.3, we review these proposed methods and give some examples of their use with biochemical data. They are intended for cross-sectional studies of individuals differing in age or some other covariate of interest. Longitudinal studies have, or should have, a quite different objective. We consider this in Section 5.4.

5.2 NONPARAMETRIC METHODS

5.2.1 Method of Healy et al.

Searching for a nonparametric procedure to avoid the assumption of a Normal distribution at each age, and recognizing that although a large number of individuals may be available overall, there will usually be only a small number in any narrow age band, Healy and coworkers (1988) proposed an alternative to the simple quantile estimator. They reasoned from the follow-

---

[1] The authors whose works we shall be describing in this chapter invariably use the word "centile" in place of "percentile." It seems to be conventional usage in studies of anthropometric data like height and weight in children and has carried over to time-dependent distributions in general.

ing premises: (1) that centiles of the distribution at any age will be smooth functions of age, and (2) that the distribution as a whole will change slowly and smoothly with age. Therefore, centiles at nearby ages share information that may be used to improve estimation at each age. Moreover, the spacing between centiles should remain fairly constant or change only slowly with age.

Given these premises, Healy et al. (1988) suggested the following steps. First, the observations should be ordered by increasing age. Next, following a procedure attributed to Cleveland (1979), the first k measurements, where k should be 5–10 percent of the total number, are regressed linearly against age, and the residuals sorted by size. Selected quantiles are computed from these and added to the expected value of the observation at the median of the k ages, and results are plotted against the median age. This procedure is repeated for the set of observations ranked 2 to $k + 1$, 3 to $k + 2$, etc., through the final set of observations ranked $(n - k + 1)$ to n. This provides a family of irregular centile plots across an age span slightly narrower than that of the original data.

The authors propose that each of these centile plots be modeled by a polynomial of degree p:

$$y_i(t) = a_{0i} + a_{1i}t + a_{2i}t^2 + \cdots + a_{pi}t^p, \tag{5.1}$$

where $y_i(t)$ denotes the smoothed ith centile at age t. Then, in an ingenious maneuver that allows for slowly changing distribution shapes at increasing ages, the coefficients a_{ji} are related to the standardized Normal deviate (z_i) corresponding to the ith centile according to another polynomial of degree q_j:

$$a_{ji} = b_{j0} + b_{j1}z_i + b_{j2}z_i^2 + \cdots + b_{jq}z_i^q, \tag{5.2}$$

where, for example, $z_i = 0$ for the 50th centile, -1.96 for the 2.5th centile, and $+1.96$ for the 97.5th centile. The degree q_j can be chosen to vary with the coefficient a_{ji}. Inserting Equation (5.2) into (5.1) produces a polynomial whose coefficients can be estimated by ordinary least squares.

There are then several adjustable constants (or parameters), k, p, and the q_j. Healy et al. (1988) considered several hypothetical cases. In the simplest, the distribution of measurements at any age is Normal with constant standard deviation. This is specified by $q_0 = 1$ and $q_j = 0$ for all $j > 0$. Then $a_{0i} = b_{00} + b_{01}z_i$, while all higher coefficients a_{1i}, a_{2i}, etc., in Equation (5.1) are independent of z_i. The centile curves are all parallel with spacings between them depending on the corresponding Normal deviates. If the distributions are Normal but with standard deviations that increase linearly with age, $q_0 = q_1 = 1$ while $q_j = 0$ for all $j > 1$. Now, $a_{1i} = b_{10} + b_{11}z_i$, so that a term in z_it appears in (5.1). Then the centile curves diverge with age. Setting $q_0 = 2$ indicates skew distributions in which the higher centiles would be spaced farther apart than expected under a Normal curve.

In short, the system offers considerable flexibility, but careful preliminary examination of the data and some experimenting is necessary to select the most appropriate values for p and the $q's$. Initial transformation of the measurement scale may help to stabilize the standard deviations across age. The shape of the distribution should not change irregularly as age increases, implying that p should probably not be more than 2. This may become a problem for wide age spans. For this situation, Pan et al. (1990) have extended the technique to separate sections of the age span, arranging for the centile curves to join smoothly across the sections.

Validation of the Healy procedure or any other method for obtaining centile charts involves counting the numbers of observations between pairs of centile curves and comparing these counts with the expected numbers through a chi-square test.

A generic problem with the use of centile charts is that of estimating the exact centile of a measurement on a new subject, assuming that the measurement lies between two adjacent curves on the chart. This can be approximated by eye, of course, but a common alternative is to compute the standard Normal deviate, or SD score, corresponding to the exact centile. Healy et al. point out that since their method assumes that any smoothed centile y_i can be expressed as a polynomial function of its corresponding standard Normal deviate z_i, the SD score of a new measurement can be calculated by solving a polynomial equation. They give an example where $p = 1$, $q_0 = 2$, and $q_1 = 1$. In this case, the ith centile curve is given by

$$y_i = (b_{00} + b_{01}z_i + b_{02}z_i^2) + (b_{10} + b_{11}z_i)t \qquad (5.3)$$

Then, given a measurement y at age t, the SD score is the solution of the quadratic equation,

$$b_{02}z^2 + (b_{01} + b_{11}t)z = y - (b_{00} + b_{10}t), \qquad (5.4)$$

where the right-hand side is the difference between the measurement and the 50th centile (i.e., that centile for which $z = 0$).

An advantage of the method of Healy et al. is that at no stage is it necessary to group the ages of the subjects into an arbitrary set of classes. This is important when the variable may be changing systematically with age, as in children. Healy (1962) has shown that such changes affect the variance, skewness, and kurtosis of a grouped distribution as compared with these moments at the central age of the group. He provided corrections for these effects when the distribution at a given age is Normal.

On the other hand, freedom from age grouping exacts a considerable cost in computer time. For example, suppose 1000 subjects at all ages have been examined, and, after sorting the measured variable by size, consecutive sets of 100 are to be regressed against the associated ages, residuals calculated and sorted for each set, and perhaps nine or ten raw centiles computed from them. A total of 900 sets of these operations would have to be carried out before the process of parameter selection and least squares curve fitting could even begin! However, an updated version of the method of Healy et al. has been implemented through the Nanostat statistical computing package, developed at the London School of Hygiene and Tropical Medicine.

An example from the clinical literature on the use of this method is given by Scott et al. (1990), who computed centile charts of maximum kidney length and depth by birth weight and head circumference in 560 newborn infants. The selected values of the parameters for all four charts were $p = 1$ (the centile curves were straight lines), $q_0 = 2$, indicating skewness in the distributions of maximum kidney length or depth for given birth weight or head circumference, and $q_1 = 1$, indicating increasing standard deviation in the kidney measurement weight as the covariate increased. Results for maximum kidney length versus birth weight are shown in Figure 5.1. In the next section we compare these results with those obtained from the same data using another nonparametric method.

5.2.2 Method of Kernel Functions

Rossiter (1991) introduced a quite different nonparametric technique for deriving centile charts. He considered the observations more generally as pairs forming a bivariate distribution over all subjects. The members of each pair might both be clinical measurements, such as height and weight, for example, but usually one will be time or the age of the subject. Accordingly, Rossiter proposed the use of a bivariate kernel function to estimate the centile curves nonparametrically.

The Harrell-Davis weighted quantile formula (Equation 2.3) discussed in Chapter 2 is an example of the use of a kernel (or weight) function to obtain a smoothed nonparametric estimate of a univariate distribution function defined at selected percentile points (see Figure 2.2). We noted there that the use of kernel functions to describe probability distributions nonparametrically has been the subject of considerable statistical research during recent years (e.g., Silverman, 1986).

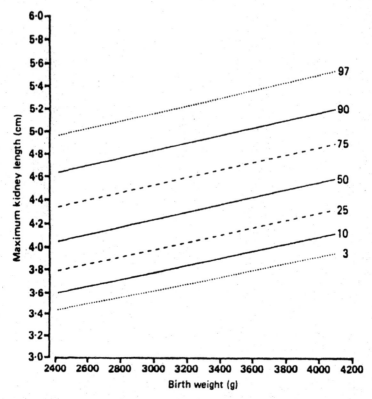

Fig. 5.1 Centile chart of maximum kidney length by birth weight using method of Healy et al. (From Scott et al., 1990, with permission.)

The general definition of a kernel estimator of a bivariate distribution $f(y,t)$ is expressed by Rossiter as

$$f(y,t) = (1/nh_i^2) \sum_{i=1}^{n} K[(y - Y_i)/h_i, (t - T_i)/h_i], \qquad (5.5)$$

where Y_i is the measured value for the ith subject and T_i is the covariate value (e.g., age), but both are scaled to have equal standard deviations; $K(y,t)$ is the kernel function, and h is a "bandwidth" which may be allowed to vary with the ith pair of values.[2] The kernel function is chosen so that for a specific pair of values y and t, it reaches its highest value when $y,t = Y_i,T_i$, and decreases toward zero as the differences $y - Y_i$ and/or $t - T_i$ increase. For example, if y_p is the estimated pth centile of the conditional distribution $f(y \mid t)$, then, as the kernel function sweeps through the entire set of observations, it should peak at that observation Y_i closest to y_p at covariate T_i closest to t. Other observation pairs receive lesser weights. Some kernel functions admit zero weights, but, in general, all observations contribute to the estimate $y_p \mid t$. Thus, we obtain a smoothing effect on the centile curves because of inclusion in the estimates of observations in the neighborhood of $y_p \mid t$ with respect to both y and t.

The kernel function is usually chosen to be a probability density function; for example, the Normal curve is a popular choice. In this case, the kernel never reaches zero and is said to have "infinite support." However, there are many possible kernel functions with similar properties, and specialists in this area agree that the exact form of the kernel function does not greatly affect the final estimate. More important is the bandwidth h because this determines the degree to which the true bivariate probability surface is smoothed when obtaining the

---

[2] As Silverman (1986) explains, the basic form of the kernel estimator of a univariate probability density function $f(x)$, namely,

$$\hat{f}(x) = (1/nh) \sum_{i=1}^{n} K[(x - X_i)/h],$$

derives from the traditional practice of estimating the shape of the distribution by grouping a sample of n observations X_i ($i = 1, \ldots, n$) into bins of constant width h to form a histogram. When the selected bin width is too large, important details of $f(x)$ may be lost; when h is too small, sampling irregularities may obscure smooth changes in $f(x)$. The use of kernel functions to smooth raw estimates of spectral densities in the frequency domain is also well known. In that literature, the kernel function is called a "spectral window" and h, the bandwidth or simply the width of the window.

estimate. A relatively small bandwidth allows an isolated modal value in the sample of data to appear as a minor peak in the estimated surface because it will not be averaged out with neighboring values that occur much less frequently. As the bandwidth increases, so does the extent of averaging, tending to smooth out irregularities in the sample frequency distribution. Clearly, a balance is needed so that fluctuations in sample frequencies that are not represented in the (unknown) true probability distribution will be smoothed away without seriously affecting the distinguishing features of the true distribution. Unfortunately, as Hill (1985) has shown, the best choice of bandwidth, in terms of minimizing the mean square error of fit to the true distribution, depends on the form of that distribution. In other words, the bandwidth is not a robust parameter.

Rossiter chose the bivariate logistic distribution (Gumbel, 1961) to use as a kernel function. The shape of this distribution, although not symmetrical, is similar to the bivariate Normal, peaking at (0,0) for two standardized variables. Unlike the Normal, it can be integrated analytically over either variable to obtain exact expressions for the conditional distribution functions. The estimated pth centile for a given value of t, say $y_p \mid t$, is determined by solving iteratively the equation

$$\frac{\sum_{i=1}^{n} c_i/(1 + \exp\{-[(y_p \mid t - Y_i)/h_i]\})}{\sum_{i=1}^{n} c_i} = p, \qquad (5.6)$$

where

$$c_i = \frac{\exp\{-[(t - T_i)/h_i]\}}{(1 + \exp\{-[(t - T_i)/h_i]\})^2}$$

is the marginal logistic distribution of t around T_i, and the function $(1 + \exp\{-[(y_p \mid t - Y_i)/h_i]\})^{-1}$ in Equation (5.6) is the cumulative logistic distribution of y, given t, at the pth centile. Rossiter found through simulation experiments that when the underlying distribution was bivariate Normal, the optimal bandwidth, using the logistic kernel, was higher for more extreme values of T_i, but more or less constant for (standardized) T_i between ± 1.5. Moreover, the optimal bandwidth was about the same for mild correlation (0.25) between the variables as it was for independent variables. In applying Rossiter's method, preliminary inspection of the data to detect outliers, and initial transformation to help stabilize variance and improve agreement with a bivariate Normal distribution, would be helpful, as is also true for other methods of calculating conditional centiles.

Rossiter applied his centile estimation technique to the data of Scott et al. relating maximum kidney length to birthweight in newborn infants, first transforming the data to logarithms. The resulting centile curves over a scatter diagram of the data appear in Figure 5.2.

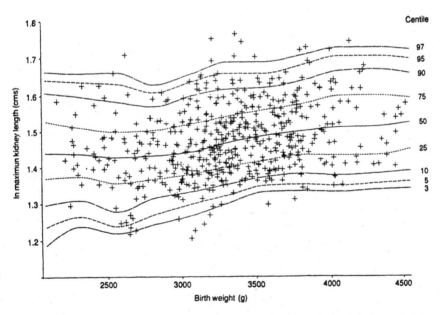

Fig. 5.2 Centile chart of maximum kidney length by birth weight using Rossiter's logistic kernel method. (From J. E. Rossiter, 1991, *Calculating centile curves using kernel density estimation methods with application to infant kidney lengths. Statistics in Medicine 10*, 1693–1701. Reprinted by permission of John Wiley & Sons, Ltd.)

The curves show some irregularity, particularly at the more extreme centiles, which the author attributed to sampling variability. However, even the smoother central centile curves appear quadratic or cubic rather than the straight lines in Figure 5.1, representing the results of using the method of Healy et al. on these data. It is inevitable that Rossiter's method will produce somewhat more irregular-looking centile curves than obtained using the method of Healy et al. since the latter requires that all the curves be fitted by polynomials of the same degree. For a quick numerical comparison by eye, we estimated the antilogs of the third and ninety-seventh centiles at 3400 g birth weight from Figure 5.2 to be 3.7 and 5.4 cms, respectively, and the same centiles from Figure 5.1 to be 3.7 and 5.3 cms.

5.3 PARAMETRIC METHODS

5.3.1 Box-Cox Transforms

In Chapter 2 we reviewed various methods recommended for transforming non-Normally distributed analytes to a new scale on which the distribution of measurements would follow a Normal curve. If the transform function achieved this objective, Normal estimators of $\xi_{0.025}$ and $\xi_{0.975}$, computed from the mean and standard deviation of the transformed measurements and then back-transformed to the original scale, would be essentially unbiased and considerably more precise than nonparametric estimators. The same kind of procedure has been recommended by van't Hof et al.(1985) and Cole (1988) for calculating reference centiles over an age span when the variable at a given age is not Normally distributed on the original measurement scale.

These authors suggested estimating for each age or age group, a Box-Cox power transform (Chapter 2, Section 2.5.2):

$$y^{(\lambda)} = \begin{cases} (y^{\lambda} - 1)/\lambda & (\lambda \neq 0), \\ \log y & (\lambda = 0). \end{cases}$$

van't Hof et al. estimated λ as the power that minimized the coefficient of skewness of the observations at a given age. These estimates were then smoothed by fitting a quadratic or straight line as appropriate across the age span. Using the smoothed values, the mean and standard deviation of the transformed measurements at every age were calculated, and smooth curves drawn through these statistics by eye. From the smoothed means and standard deviations, Normal estimators for selected centiles were calculated and back-transformed to produce centile curves on the original measurement scale.

Cole determined the maximum likelihood estimate (mle) of λ. As Box and Cox noted, the mle of λ minimizes the variance of the scaled variable $f^{(\lambda)} = y^{(\lambda)}/\dot{y}^{\lambda-1}$, where $\dot{y}$ is the geometric mean of the measurement on the original scale. Cole preferred to minimize the variance of $g^{(\lambda)} = f^{(\lambda)}/\dot{y} = y^{(\lambda)}/\dot{y}^{\lambda}$, which also leads to the mle of λ. His reason is that $g^{(\lambda)}$ is a dimensionless number whose standard deviation is similar to the coefficient of variation of the original measurement (exactly the same for $\lambda = 0$) and is likely to remain fairly constant across the age span. He uses the minimization technique referred to in Chapter 2, where, in this case, the log of the variance of $g^{(\lambda)}$ is computed for $\lambda = -1, 0, +1$, respectively, and the minimum of the quadratic curve through these points is the mle of λ.

From this estimate of λ for each age group, and assuming that $y^{\hat{\lambda}}$ is Normally distributed, Cole computes two other statistics for the age group. First, M, the median of the measurement on the original scale, calculated as $v^{1/\hat{\lambda}}$ ($\hat{\lambda} \neq 0$), where v is the mean of $y^{\hat{\lambda}}$. For $\hat{\lambda} = 0$, $v = \dot{y}$, and $M = \exp(v)$. Then, S, the standard deviation of $g^{(\lambda)}$, computed as $\epsilon/(\hat{\lambda}\dot{y}^{\hat{\lambda}})$ ($\hat{\lambda} \neq 0$), where ϵ is the standard deviation of $y^{\hat{\lambda}}$, or, for $\hat{\lambda} = 0$, $S = \epsilon$. The assumption that the power transform has succeeded in producing a Normal distribution at a given age should be tested as in the examples of Chapter 2, computing not only a goodness-of-fit test like the Shapiro-Wilk test but also the coefficients of skewness and kurtosis.

The quantities $\hat{\lambda}_j$ (which Cole calls L_j), M_j, and S_j for the jth age group are plotted against the midpoint age of the group.

These plots are converted to smooth curves $L(t)$, $M(t)$, and $S(t)$ by eye, or by fitting an appropriate polynomial or special mathematical model. Cole devotes considerable attention to interpeting the shapes of these functions in particular applications, especially $L(t)$, which indicates changes with age in the shape of the original distribution of measurements, and $S(t)$ which, as noted earlier, is like the coefficient of variation on the original scale.

The user is likely to be more interested in the final centile curves and a formula for computing the SD score (standard Normal deviate) for a new measurement. The curve for the 100α-th centile, assuming $L(t) \neq 0$, is given by

$$C_{100\alpha}(t) = M(t)[1 + L(t)S(t)z_\alpha]^{1/L(t)}, \tag{5.7}$$

where z_α is the corresponding standard Normal deviate. If $L(t)$ happens to equal zero, $C_{100\alpha}(t) = M(t)\exp[S(t)z_\alpha]$. The SD for a new measurement Y at age T is computed as

$$Z = \frac{[Y/M(T)]^{L(T)} - 1}{L(T)S(T)} \tag{5.8}$$

The paper by Cole was presented at a meeting of the Royal Statistical Society and followed, as is the custom, by a vigorous published discussion. Cole acknowledged that a drawback of his method is the need to subdivide the data into age groups in order to estimate the power transform. During the discussion, P. Green suggested that this problem, and indeed the entire process of separate estimation of the power transform and related statistics in each age group, could be avoided using the estimation procedure called *penalized maximum likelihood* (e.g., Silverman, 1986, p. 110 ff). This was later followed up in a joint publication by Cole and Green (1992). This method leads directly to estimated smooth functions $L(t)$, $S(t)$, and $M(t)$ in the form of cubic splines.

The need to group ages is not a serious problem when the measured variable is changing only slowly across the age span, as is true for many biochemical analytes among adults. It would be more significant, of course, in studying changes during childhood, depending on how narrow the groups can be made without too greatly reducing the number of subjects in each group. With respect to the use of centile curves in monitoring an individual, as opposed to initial evaluation, S. Chinn, the leading discussant of Cole's paper, remarked that centile curves should not be used for this purpose, much as the one-dimensional cross-sectional reference range should not be used for interpreting repeated measurements from one subject. Instead, Chinn saw the need for "conditional standards," based on longitudinal data, from which the distribution of second measurements, given the first, could be estimated. We discuss these in Section 5.4.

Finally, Cole mentioned the sensitivity of the estimate λ to outlying observations and recommended recomputing the mle of λ once or twice, excluding extreme high and low observations. In this regard, Healy noted during the discussion that failure to achieve a Normal distribution in a given age group could lead to serious bias in the estimation of extreme centiles or SD scores where most of the clinical interest lies.

5.3.2 Other Methods

The three methods reviewed above (two nonparametric, one parametric) for deriving covariate (usually, age)-dependent centile curves were all recently published. More experience with clinical data, including biochemical analytes, will determine the popularity of each among biostatisticians, clinicians, and clinical laboratorians. At this point, we turn to a simpler procedure that has been described recently in two reports, one by Isaacs et al. (1983) on determining reference ranges by age for serum immunoglobulins IgG, IgA, and IgM in preschool children, the second by P. Royston (1991), a more detailed statistical guideline to constructing time-specific reference ranges. Royston includes as examples increasing serum cholesterol with age in women and declining fetal triglycerides with gestational age.

Although these two papers differ somewhat in methodological details, both follow the same general procedure.

This procedure features one characteristic resembling Rossiter's approach, namely, that the entire sample of n paired observations is approached as a unified bivariate distribution rather than subdividing the sample into consecutive sets, as in Healy's method, or grouping the covariate (e.g., age) into narrow bands as Cole suggested. The procedure is parametric, however, for it seeks to find a single transform function, if needed, to convert the conditional distribution of the measured variable at any age to Normal form.

Before and after transformation, a polynomial of appropriate degree is fitted through the scatter diagram of paired values. The residuals are tested for conformity to a Normal distribution, using the Shapiro-Wilk test for large samples (J. P. Royston, 1982) as well as plotting the residuals on Normal probability paper and computing coefficients of skewness and kurtosis (however, see later discussion). Isaacs et al. chose the logarithmic transform for IgA and IgM, but the square root for IgG. Royston decided at the beginning to search no farther than the log or $\log(x + C)$ scales and finds one or the other of these successful in his examples.

The fitted polynomial regression of analyte value (after transformation) against age represents the estimated 50th centile curve on the transformed scale. The variability of residuals about this curve is crucial to the determination of reliable reference ranges with age, assuming that, taken as a whole, the residuals conform to a Normal distribution. Often, the standard deviation of the residual depends on the age of the subject, and this will have to be accounted for in estimating the centile limits at any age. Isaacs et al. recommended grouping the residuals into, say, eight age brackets and fitting a linear or quadratic curve to describe changes in the standard deviations with age. Royston suggested dividing the residuals into thirds, bounded by the 33rd and 67th age percentiles, and testing the ratio of the standard deviations of upper and lower groups through an F-test. If indicated, a line may be plotted through the standard deviations of each group.

More recently, Altman (1993) has pointed out that if the residuals are time- (e.g., age-) dependent, then probability plots and tests of skewness or kurtosis should be carried out on the standardized residuals (i.e., the residuals divided by their respective standard deviations). Altman noted that if, in fact, the residuals are Normally distributed, their age-dependent standard deviations can be determined without arbitrary grouping into age bands. Instead, the absolute values of the residuals should be plotted individually against age and fitted by a linear or quadratic curve as seems reasonable. Then, multiplying the regression coefficients by $\sqrt{\pi/2}$, the resulting equation will represent the standard deviation of the original (signed) values as a function of age.

Normal estimators of the reference limits (and other centiles if desired) at a given age are obtained from the estimated 50th centile plus and minus the appropriate multiple of the standard deviation computed from its regression curve, followed by back-transformation of the result to the original scale. Joining these estimators produces the desired centile curves. Figure 5.3 illustrates Royston's estimated 5th, 50th, and 95th centile curves over age for serum cholesterol in women.

Clearly, all these methods of deriving age- (or other covariate) dependent reference limits involve a degree of statistical judgment throughout the process supported by careful preliminary inspection of the data for such problems as obvious measurement errors, apparent outliers, possible misidentifications, bias or rounding in reported ages. With respect to biochemical analytes in adults, the simpler methods just described should produce reliable results, although the search for Normalizing functions might be widened to include the general Box-Cox power transforms. P. Royston (1991) points out that if the graph of standard deviations of residuals against age does not conform to a low-degree polynomial, even a straight line, another, more complex, method of deriving centile curves is probably needed. This is the critical justification for using a simpler procedure, besides, of course, the final test of whether the proportions of observations between estimated centiles agree reasonably well with expected values.

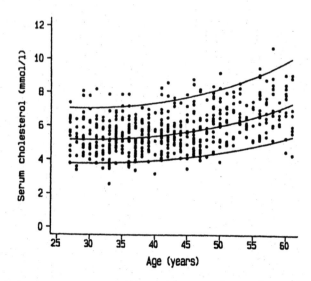

Fig. 5.3 Estimated 5th, 50th, and 95th centiles of serum cholesterol in women, by age. (From P. Royston, 1991, Constructing time-specific reference ranges. *Statistics in Medicine 10*, 675–690. Reprinted by permission of John Wiley & Sons, Ltd.)

5.3.3 Example: Derivation of Age-Adjusted Reference Limits for Serum Prostate–Specific Antigen

Serum prostate–specific antigen (PSA) is widely recognized as a sensitive biochemical indicator of the recurrence of prostate cancer following treatment (e.g., prostatectomy or radiation therapy). It has also been recently approved by the Food and Drug Administration for initial detection of this disease, particularly when combined with digital rectal examination (DRE) and ultrasound or magnetic resonance imaging. In this application, PSA is known to be nonspecific for prostate cancer because it is also increased in the presence of benign hypertrophy of the prostate and other nonmalignant diseases of the prostate.

As part of National Prostate Week in October, 1993, men in the Charlottesville and Albemarle County area of Virginia were invited by newspaper and television notices placed by the University of Virginia Department of Urology to come for a free prostate screening. A total of 371 men responded. Each participant completed a questionnaire regarding family history of prostatic disease and urological symptoms he may have experienced. In addition, each subject underwent a DRE performed by a urologist and had a blood sample drawn for serum PSA determination. All blood samples were drawn prior to any prostatic manipulation. The serum PSA concentration was determined with the Tosoh Medics PSA assay (Tosoh Medics Inc., Foster City, Calif). The manufacturer's reference range for this assay is 0.47–3.04 μg/L.

All participants with abnormal results from either the DRE or PSA were urged to have further evaluation at the University or their private urologists. The outcomes of these evaluations were assessed through follow-up questionnaires approximately 6 months after the initial screening. Only one subject was discovered to have prostatic adenocarcinoma, and his data were excluded from further analysis. Also excluded were PSA results from six men over the age of 80 and one 73-year old subject whose PSA was 27.4 μg/L, an extreme value more than twice as high as the next highest result. This patient was found to have an unusually enlarged prostate, but multiple prostate biopsies were negative for adenocarcinoma. The PSA data from the remaining 363 patients are listed in Appendix 5.1.

Our main purpose in analyzing these data is to illustrate the use of the simpler methods suggested by P. Royston and Altman for deriving age-related reference limits. However, we should point out that these data were obtained from subjects who selected themselves for inclusion rather than from a random sample of the population of men in the region. We might anticipate that a greater proportion of the men in a self-selected rather than a random sample would have experienced early symptoms of prostate hyperplasia and would in fact show higher PSA values. The potential bias of a self-selected sample is well known to epidemiologists. Full investigation of this possibility would require analysis of the questionnaire information.

However, we can compare our estimated reference limits with those obtained recently by Oesterling et al. (1993), who did carry out a random sampling study of PSA in subjects with no evidence of prostate cancer. This comparison is presented at the end of this section.

As expected, the original data were highly asymmetric, nor was log PSA Normally distributed over all ages (Shapiro-Wilk statistic $W = 0.964$, $P < 0.0001$, using J. P. Royston's normalizing transformation for large samples). Instead, a linear relationship was observed between log PSA and age of subject; second- and higher-order coefficients were not significantly different from zero. The regression equation was

$$\log_e \text{PSA} = 0.0310 \text{ (age)} - 1.770, \tag{5.9}$$

for ages between 28 and 79 years.

Within the age decades 40–49, 50–59, 60–69 and 70–79, residuals from the fitted model [Equation (5.9)] were Normally distributed but showed significant heteroscedasticity with higher standard deviations among older individuals. To avoid age-grouping, the method of Altman was applied, modeling the regression of the absolute values of the residuals against age. A linear model was sufficient. Multiplying the slope and intercept by $\sqrt{\pi/2}$, the final equation was

$$\text{SD (log PSA)} = 0.00777 \text{ (age)} + 0.3734 \tag{5.10}$$

The age-standardized residuals, obtained by dividing each residual by the calculated SD (log PSA) for that subject's age (Equation 5.10) were found to be Normally distributed, justifying the use of Altman's procedure. Since only upper reference limits for PSA are clinically important, the 90th and 95th centile points were estimated from the mean log PSA for that age as given by Equation (5.9), adding 1.28 (90th centile) or 1.645 (95th centile) times the SD for that age. The resulting curves (after back-transformation to original scale) are shown in Figure 5.4. Eighteen PSA values (5.0 percent) lie outside the 95th centile curve, whereas 37 values (10.2 percent) lie outside the 90th centile curve, confirming the validity of the Normal estimators for these data.

In the study by Oesterling et al., a sample of almost 4000 white males 40–79 years of age without a history of prostate cancer was randomly chosen from a population of over 100,000 in Olmsted County, Minnesota. Of this sample, slightly over 2000 men (55%) agreed to participate in the prostate evaluation. There was, therefore, an element of self-selection here, but comparison of the medical records of these individuals with those in the sample who did not agree to participate did not reveal any significant differences. The Tandem-R PSA assay (Hybri-

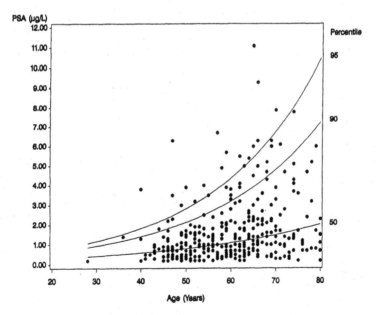

Fig. 5.4 Estimated 50th, 90th, and 95th centiles of serum prostate-specific antigen (PSA).

tech Inc., San Diego, Calif.) was used, for which the manufacturer's reference range is 0.0–4.0 µg/L, slightly wider than that of the assay employed in the Virginia study.

Oesterling et al. found the PSA results to be logNormally distributed (whether over all ages or within each age decade is not clear), and the regression of log PSA against age was computed. Then, results were grouped into 10-year age groups, and, apparently, the observed percentiles of log PSA in each group, rather than Normal estimators, were used to estimate centile limits at the midpoint of the age group. The points for each centile were joined to produce smooth curves. Since no mention was made of any analysis of the relationship between the standard deviation of residuals and age, it was probably just as well that observed percentiles were used as estimators within each age group, but clearly a more precise analysis of the data would have been preferable. With these caveats in mind, including the difference between the analytical procedures employed, Table 5.1 lists the estimated 50th, 90th, and 95th centile points for ages 45, 55, 65, and 75 years obtained in each of these two studies. The centiles for the Minnesota study (Oesterling et al.) were estimated from the published smooth curves across all ages (Fig. 1, p. 863).

The median results of the two studies are quite comparable at all ages, as are the 90th and 95th centile limits for men in their 40s. At ages of 55 and older, however, the upper centile

Table 5.1 Estimated 50th, 90th, and 95th Centiles of Serum PSA at Four Ages in Two Studies

	45		55		65		75	
	Va.	Minn.	Va.	Minn.	Va.	Minn.	Va.	Minn.
50th	0.69	0.7	0.93	1.0	1.27	1.3	1.74	1.7
90th	1.73	1.7	2.61	2.4	3.92	3.4	5.90	4.8
95th	2.26	2.3	3.50	3.1	5.43	4.4	8.41	6.2

limits from the Virginia study are increasingly higher than those from the Minnesota study. This may indicate the effects of self-selection bias since men at these ages are more likely to have experienced symptoms of prostate disease, and those who volunteer for PSA assay are perhaps more likely to show higher values.

5.4 LONGITUDINAL DATA; CONDITIONAL CHANGES

Although longitudinal (i.e., repeated) measurements of biochemical constituents have occasionally been used to calculate time-dependent reference centiles (e.g., O'Leary et al., 1991), they are not well suited to this task. The problem lies in the serial correlation of successive observations in an individual whose circulating level of the analyte is continually changing with time. A random sample of individuals during this time of change will, on the average, exhibit a course of increasing (or decreasing) values that may be fitted by a polynomial or some other mathematical function, and this average curve could be used to estimate approximately the 50th centile. However, individual analyte concentrations will generally be changing at either a faster or slower rate than the average. In the former case, residual deviations from the average will always be positive; in the latter, always negative. In either case, within-subject residuals will be correlated. The standard deviation of residuals across individuals will tend to be larger and the resulting centile curves more widely separated than those obtained from cross-sectional data. Even so, a higher than expected proportion of observations would likely be found to exceed the highest centile curve or fall below the lowest curve. This was noted (and correctly attributed to serial correlation) by O'Leary et al. (1991) in their longitudinal study of changes in reproductive hormones during normal pregnancy. Three blood samples were taken from each woman, once during each trimester. In this study, 5 and 95 percent as well as 50 percent centile curves were calculated.

Centile curves derived from longitudinal data according to a method appropriate for cross-sectional data will bias the interpretation of a single measurement in a new individual. Conversely, however, repeated measurements from a large sample of subjects during a period of change in the analyte *are* required for the development of *conditional* reference values to be used for interpreting the change in a second measurement in a new individual given his or her initial value. As mentioned earlier, S. Chinn pointed this out during the discussion following Cole's paper (1988). Cameron (1980) provides an example in the derivation of "conditional standards" for growth in height of British children, based on two measurements approximately a year apart. Adjusting for minor deviations in the actual time intervals between "annual" measurements, Cameron determined the slope, intercept, and average standard deviation of residuals characterizing a linear change in height from age t to age $t + 1$ in children between 5 and 15 years of age. As would be expected, the average correlation between measurements of a child's height from one year to the next was extremely high, greater than 0.94 at any age.

5.4.1 Regression to the Mean

Repeated measurements of biochemical analytes in blood during childhood (and especially during infancy) would be uncommon because of the invasive nature of blood sampling. Nevertheless, the development of conditional reference values in blood chemistries during growth and other special times of change is probably a clinically useful area of investigation. It faces a fundamental difficulty, however, that does not arise in repeated measurements of such variables as height in children. This is the problem of *regression to the mean*.

The definition of this statistical phenomenon traces back to studies by Galton in the last century on the relationship between the heights of sons and the heights of fathers, but the underlying causes of regression to the mean as seen in repeated measurements of blood constituents are quite different. They relate to the analytical and biological components of within-person variability.

Suppose that measurement errors or random time-to-time fluctuations in the circulating levels of an analyte within an individual did not exist, and that all persons remained in steady state during the interval between two measurements. Then, those individuals whose values at initial measurement were relatively high, say, in the upper decile of the population, would remain in exactly the same position on repeated measurement. The correlation between first and second measurements would be unity, and the only variation would be that among individual mean values. The data of Cameron (1980) show that when the time interval between measurements is short, measurement error is extremely small, and random within-person fluctuations are absent, the observed correlation can be very close to unity.

For biochemical analytes, random within-person variability can be substantial, causing the correlation between repeated measurements to become attenuated. As a result, regression to the mean will induce repeated observations, given initial readings in the highest decile, to spread out more widely than might be expected solely from the unequal effects of any systematic physiological change.

This is an especially serious problem in clinical studies that measure the effect of intervention to reduce the level of a physiological variable (e.g., blood pressure or serum cholesterol). Such studies usually choose to intervene only in subjects whose initial measurements are above some defined critical level. Unless matched controls are included, it may be difficult to determine what proportion of the observed change after treatment is attributable to the intervention and what to regression to the mean that would occur in the absence of any treatment effect. James (1973) and Davis (1976) discuss statistical methods of resolving this issue in uncontrolled studies, but stress the importance of including controls to avoid the problem.

A clear example of the importance of regression to the mean in interpreting conditional changes in blood chemistries may be found in a recent French study of changes during childhood (Spyckerelle et al., 1992). In France, the social security system accords family members the opportunity to receive complete medical examinations including clinical laboratory tests every 5 years, beginning at 4 years of age. As a means of early detection of high-risk individuals, it would be desirable to estimate from such data the probability that a child of a given age whose analyte value falls within a high range would exhibit a value 5 years later in the same range.

Spyckerelle et al. examined such changes in cholesterol, uric acid, and blood glucose in children from 4 to 16 years of age at initial examination. They found that for cholesterol and uric acid, only 40–50 percent of the children in the upper two deciles at first examination remained in that range after 5 years, the percentage varying somewhat with the gender and initial age of the child. For glucose, the percentage remaining in this high range averaged about 30 percent. The average correlation between first and second measurements was 0.5–0.6 for cholesterol and uric acid, but only about 0.3 for glucose. To what extent can these results be explained by statistical regression to the mean?

The general theory underlying an analysis of the data to try to answer this question may be outlined as follows. Assume that the measurements of a given analyte (or some transformation of them to another scale) are Normally distributed across the population of interest (e.g., girls or boys of a given age at first observation). Let x_i and y_i represent the first and second measurements, respectively, of the ith child. Suppose each of these variables has been reduced to standard form by subtracting the mean and dividing by the standard deviation. Let the upper 20 percent of the distribution of x_i be defined by some cutpoint, x_c; in the Spyckerelle study, x_c was the sample quantile $Q_{0.80}$. The conditional distribution of y_i, given $x_i > x_c$ (all now in standard form), is given by the following formula (e.g.,

Moran, 1968, p. 316), omitting the subscript i:

$$f(y \mid x > x_c) = \{2\pi[1 - \Phi(x_c)](1 - \rho^2)^{1/2}\}^{-1}$$

$$\int_{x_c}^{\infty} \exp\left[-\frac{1}{2}\frac{x^2 - 2\rho xy + y^2}{1 - \rho^2}\right] dx \qquad (5.11)$$

where

$$1 - \Phi(x_c) = (2\pi)^{-1/2} \int_{x_c}^{\infty} \exp(-\tfrac{1}{2}x^2)\, dx,$$

and ρ is the correlation between x and y.

Using integration by parts, Moran also gives formulas for the mean and variance of y given $x > x_c$. The latter formula is particularly instructive:

$$\text{Var}(y \mid x > x_c) = 1 - \rho^2 W(W - x_c), \qquad (5.12)$$

where $W = [\exp(-x_c^2/2)]/\{(2\pi)^{1/2}[1 - \Phi(x_c)]\}$.

The smaller the correlation between x and y, the larger will be the variance of y given $x > x_c$, and thus the wider will be the distribution of these second measurements. For example, choosing $x_c = 0.84$, the 80th percentile of the standard Normal distribution, and setting $\rho = 0.9$, we obtain $\text{Var}(y \mid x > 0.84)$ = 0.3673, or SD = 0.606. For $\rho = 0.5$, SD $(y \mid x > 0.84)$ = 0.897, or 48 percent higher.

Given the average correlations between first and second measurements observed by Spyckerelle et al., it is not surprising that, when first measurements were in the upper 80 percent range, they found a high proportion of second measurements of cholesterol and uric acid below this level, and an even higher proportion in glucose.

The general conclusion we reach concerning the development of clinically useful conditional reference standards for biochemical analytes is that it is probably not practical except in cases where analytic variance and biological within-subject variance form a very small proportion of total variance. On the other hand, the possibility of detecting in early childhood individuals facing a high risk of developing serious disease in later life (e.g., coronary heart disease) is a powerful inducement to the study of repeated measurements of selected analytes. The search for such individuals demands measurement at more than two occasions, at least three or four, winnowing out those whose values are not consistently above the selected cutpoint.

To sum up, we have cautioned against the use of longitudinal biochemical data in two areas: (1) to derive group-based time-dependent centile curves during periods of rapid change, such as pregnancy, and (2) to derive conditional reference values for periods of relatively slow change, such as childhood. In the first case, the problem is high serial correlation between observations, due to driving deterministic factors that overwhelm the random effects of measurement error or day-to-day biological fluctuations. In these circumstances, centile curves should be derived from cross-sectional observations. In the second case, the problem is low serial correlation because the systematic changes occur at much lower rates, allowing random effects to exert greater influence on the observed variation.

Random effects become most important when longitudinal biochemical data are analyzed to detect person-specific changes from steady state. This will be the topic of Chapter 7.

APPENDIX 5.1   AGE AND PSA MEASUREMENTS FROM
                A STUDY OF 371 MEN AT THE
                UNIVERSITY OF VIRGINIA (ONE
                OUTLIER, ONE CONFIRMED CANCER,
                AND DATA FROM SIX MEN OVER 80
                YEARS OLD DELETED)

Data begins on p. 179.

OBS	AGE	PSA
1	28	0.20
2	36	1.40
3	40	1.30
4	40	0.20
5	40	3.80
6	41	0.50
7	41	0.30
8	41	0.30
9	42	0.50
10	43	0.90
11	43	0.70
12	43	1.00
13	43	0.30
14	43	0.70
15	43	0.60
16	44	0.80
17	44	1.80
18	45	0.70
19	45	0.20
20	45	0.40
21	45	1.40
22	45	0.70
23	45	0.90
24	46	0.70
25	46	0.90
26	46	0.40
27	46	0.80
28	46	0.50
29	46	1.20
30	46	0.20
31	46	1.70
32	46	1.30
33	46	0.20
34	46	0.90
35	46	0.40
36	46	0.70
37	46	2.20
38	47	0.80
39	47	6.30
40	47	0.40
41	47	3.50
42	47	0.80
43	47	0.80
44	47	2.30
45	47	0.50
46	47	0.30
47	47	0.30
48	47	0.70
49	47	0.90
50	48	0.40

OBS	AGE	PSA
51	48	0.70
52	48	1.00
53	48	1.00
54	48	0.30
55	48	1.00
56	49	1.60
57	49	0.40
58	49	0.80
59	49	1.10
60	49	0.50
61	49	1.50
62	49	0.40
63	49	3.00
64	49	0.40
65	49	0.20
66	49	0.30
67	49	0.80
68	49	0.90
69	50	0.70
70	50	0.30
71	50	3.90
72	50	0.40
73	50	1.00
74	50	0.40
75	50	1.40
76	50	0.50
77	50	0.30
78	50	1.10
79	50	1.70
80	50	0.30
81	50	1.10
82	50	1.50
83	51	0.20
84	51	0.60
85	51	0.20
86	51	0.60
87	51	0.90
88	51	0.60
89	51	0.60
90	51	0.70
91	51	0.50
92	51	2.00
93	51	1.60
94	51	0.30
95	52	0.40
96	52	1.90
97	52	0.20
98	52	1.50
99	52	1.60
100	52	0.40

OBS	AGE	PSA
101	52	1.10
102	52	3.20
103	52	0.70
104	52	0.40
105	52	1.30
106	53	0.20
107	53	0.90
108	53	0.40
109	53	0.40
110	53	1.60
111	53	1.20
112	53	1.90
113	53	1.00
114	53	0.40
115	53	0.90
116	53	0.90
117	54	4.00
118	54	0.90
119	54	0.80
120	54	0.60
121	54	1.80
122	54	1.00
123	54	1.50
124	54	0.90
125	54	2.50
126	54	1.00
127	54	0.20
128	55	3.50
129	55	0.70
130	55	0.40
131	55	0.70
132	55	0.40
133	55	1.00
134	55	1.40
135	55	1.00
136	55	0.80
137	56	2.40
138	56	1.20
139	56	0.20
140	56	0.70
141	56	1.50
142	56	1.80
143	56	0.90
144	56	1.30
145	56	1.40
146	56	0.70
147	56	1.00
148	57	0.50
149	57	0.60
150	57	0.40

OBS	AGE	PSA
151	57	0.40
152	57	0.50
153	57	0.50
154	57	6.70
155	57	0.30
156	57	0.60
157	57	1.00
158	58	0.40
159	58	1.50
160	58	1.30
161	58	0.90
162	58	2.10
163	58	0.40
164	58	4.90
165	58	0.30
166	58	1.90
167	58	2.60
168	59	0.50
169	59	1.00
170	59	1.80
171	59	0.90
172	59	0.70
173	59	2.10
174	59	0.60
175	59	0.60
176	59	1.00
177	59	3.90
178	59	0.70
179	59	1.70
180	59	0.40
181	59	5.70
182	59	2.00
183	60	0.70
184	60	3.80
185	60	0.50
186	60	3.50
187	60	2.80
188	60	0.90
189	60	2.20
190	60	0.60
191	60	0.50
192	60	0.40
193	60	3.30
194	60	2.80
195	60	0.60
196	61	2.10
197	61	0.30
198	61	0.50
199	61	0.50
200	61	1.50

OBS	AGE	PSA
201	61	1.30
202	61	1.40
203	61	3.10
204	61	0.50
205	61	0.30
206	61	1.00
207	61	0.70
208	61	0.70
209	61	0.50
210	62	0.70
211	62	1.30
212	62	4.10
213	62	3.90
214	62	3.20
215	62	1.00
216	62	1.80
217	62	0.20
218	62	0.40
219	62	0.90
220	62	5.50
221	62	0.90
222	63	1.00
223	63	5.00
224	63	1.10
225	63	0.90
226	63	2.10
227	63	0.60
228	63	0.40
229	63	1.00
230	63	1.00
231	63	0.20
232	63	0.50
233	63	1.70
234	63	1.80
235	63	0.70
236	64	1.40
237	64	2.40
238	64	0.80
239	64	0.50
240	64	1.30
241	64	2.20
242	64	2.60
243	64	0.60
244	64	1.50
245	64	2.70
246	64	5.40
247	65	0.70
248	65	6.00
249	65	4.50
250	65	1.80

OBS	AGE	PSA
251	65	0.80
252	65	1.20
253	65	2.20
254	65	1.40
255	65	0.80
256	65	4.50
257	65	3.00
258	65	2.30
259	65	1.00
260	65	2.40
261	65	1.00
262	65	11.10
263	66	3.30
264	66	0.40
265	66	0.50
266	66	0.70
267	66	1.20
268	66	9.30
269	66	0.40
270	66	3.30
271	66	6.30
272	66	0.40
273	66	1.00
274	66	1.00
275	66	1.40
276	66	2.00
277	66	5.00
278	66	2.30
279	66	1.10
280	67	2.20
281	67	2.30
282	67	1.10
283	67	2.00
284	67	1.50
285	67	3.60
286	67	1.10
287	67	2.00
288	67	2.70
289	68	1.40
290	68	4.30
291	68	4.70
292	68	1.00
293	68	1.60
294	68	0.40
295	68	2.10
296	68	5.20
297	68	1.00
298	69	1.60
299	69	1.60
300	69	0.40

OBS	AGE	PSA
301	69	0.50
302	69	6.30
303	69	2.30
304	69	1.60
305	69	3.00
306	69	1.00
307	69	6.00
308	69	2.20
309	70	3.30
310	70	1.10
311	70	1.70
312	70	7.90
313	70	0.60
314	70	3.90
315	70	0.30
316	70	1.90
317	70	1.40
318	71	1.70
319	71	6.10
320	71	2.50
321	71	0.30
322	71	1.00
323	72	0.40
324	72	1.40
325	72	4.70
326	72	0.40
327	72	0.90
328	72	2.80
329	72	1.00
330	73	0.40
331	73	1.30
332	73	0.60
333	73	0.30
334	74	7.80
335	74	1.30
336	74	5.10
337	74	1.40
338	74	0.70
339	74	3.70
340	74	4.10
341	74	4.30
342	74	1.50
343	75	0.20
344	75	3.60
345	75	1.70
346	76	1.20
347	76	0.70
348	76	1.10
349	76	1.00
350	77	0.70

OBS	AGE	PSA
351	77	2.40
352	77	4.70
353	78	5.20
354	78	0.80
355	78	3.20
356	79	1.70
357	79	0.80
358	79	6.00
359	80	0.70
360	80	1.10
361	80	2.30
362	80	1.50
363	80	0.20

6

COMPARISON OF WITHIN-SUBJECT AND AMONG-SUBJECTS VARIANCES

6.1 INTRODUCTION

In Chapter 3, we alluded briefly to subject-specific reference ranges and their use in monitoring the health status of individuals. Similarly, in Chapter 1, we spoke of decision levels that for some purposes, such as prevention of coronary heart disease, have become the new reference values, replacing conventional reference ranges. Increasing emphasis on prevention or early detection of disease necessarily involves monitoring individuals while they are in apparently good health or, at least, in remission of disease after treatment.

Statistically speaking, the key element in subject-specific ranges, decision levels, and patient monitoring is within-subject variance, that is, variation from time to time in the quantity being measured in one individual. In contrast, the cross-sectional reference range is largely influenced by among-subjects variance, reflecting human diversity in genetic background, environment, and behavior at the time the analyte is measured. In this chapter, we show how the ratio of within-subject to among-subjects variance can help to distinguish the appropriate clinical uses of cross-sectional and subject-specific reference ranges.

It is only quite recently that concern with within-subject variation has reached the level of general medical practice. This has to do in part with the rapid development during the last 15 years or so of biochemical tumor markers for use in early detection of site-specific cancers and monitoring for possible recurrence after initial treatment. In addition, the greatly increased public awareness of cholesterol and other lipids in the blood as early warning signals of future coronary heart disease has led to greater acceptance of routine monitoring of biochemical analytes. However, the literature shows recognition of the existence and potential importance of within-subject variation going back at least to the 1950s.

A pioneer in developing the concept of biochemical individuality was Roger Williams, whose book on the subject (1956) demonstrated that the "average" person whose biochemical measurements were all within the "normal range" was a fiction seldom, if ever, found in real life. Virtually all apparently healthy individuals would be found outside this range in one or more biochemical analytes. With this as his main thesis, Williams tended to downplay within-person variation, but he did undertake repeated sampling in small groups of subjects (e.g., 1955) and noted those who showed unusual variability in certain biochemical quantities.

More relevant to the subject of this chapter is a paper by Schneider (1960), remarkable for the clinical literature of the time, that distinguished within-subject, among-subjects, and analytical variances as separate components of the variance in single-sample cross-sectional distributions. The following quotation from Schneider's article is appropriate here:

> No matter how finely we restrict a group of healthy persons by age, sex and other criteria, and no matter how narrowly we restrict our observations in the same individual with respect to time of day, relation to meals and other physiologic conditions, in general we are left with unexplained variability from time to time and from person to person.

Schneider expressed these components of variance in a common statistical format,

$$\sigma = (\sigma_b^2 + \sigma_w^2 + \sigma_a^2)^{1/2}, \tag{6.1}$$

where σ is the standard deviation of the cross-sectional distribution of an analyte; σ_b^2, the among-subjects variance (the variance of the subjects' "true" mean values during the course of the study); σ_w^2, the within-subject variance; and σ_a^2, the "within-run" analytical variance, defined as the variance of replicate measurements from a single specimen.

As noted in Chapter 2, Section 2.5.1, the single-sample cross-sectional distribution cannot be deconstructed to allow calculation of these components separately. This requires an investigation in which a number of reference subjects are sampled repeatedly during a time span, and biochemical analyses of separate portions (aliquots) from each specimen are performed. When such a study has been completed and analysis of the data has provided separate estimates of σ_b^2, σ_w^2, and σ_a^2, these can then be summed to estimate the cross-sectional variance of single determinations from subjects of the same population. Thus, Equation (6.1) represents an application of components of variance, not a basis for estimating them.

The simplest, and standard, model for estimating these components is derived as follows. Supposing n subjects, each sampled at t successive times with p replicate determinations made on each specimen, let x_{ijk} ($i = 1, \ldots, n; j = 1, \ldots, t;$ $k = 1, \ldots, p$) be the measurement obtained from the kth aliquot of the jth specimen from the i-th subject. Then, a linear additive model for the expected value of x_{ijk} may be written,

$$E(x_{ijk}) = \mu + (\mu_i - \mu) + (\mu_{j(i)} - \mu_i) + (\mu_{k(j,i)} - \mu_{j(i)}),$$

$$(6.2)$$

where μ is the (unknown) mean concentration of the analyte in all possible specimens that could be secured over the time span of the study from the population of reference subjects; μ_i, the mean in the ith subject; $\mu_{j(i)}$, the actual concentration of the analyte in the jth specimen from the ith subject; and $\mu_{k(j,i)}$, the true concentration in the kth aliquot of the jth specimen from the ith subject. We presume that all subjects, specimens, and aliquots have been randomly selected from their respective populations whose mean values are μ, μ_i, and $\mu_{j(i)}$. For example, the t specimens from the ith subject are assumed to be a random selection of all possible specimens from this subject during the time span of the study.[1] Then, the deviations expressed in Equation (6.2) [e.g., $(\mu_{j(i)} - \mu_i)$] are random "effects" whose distributions have zero means and variances σ_b^2, σ_w^2,

---

[1] We assume implicitly that the subject is in the same "steady state" at each sampling time (see Section 6.2).

and σ_a^2, respectively. As indicated, these effects are nested within a hierarchy. The method of estimating the variances, called a *random effects* (or *components*) analysis of variance, is described in many texts on statistical inference (e.g., Milliken and Johnson, 1984, Chaps. 18–21) and included in comprehensive statistical computing packages such as SAS, BMDP, SPSS, and others. Unequal numbers of samples per subject are easily accommodated, as seen in Table 6.1, illustrating the standard format of a random effects analysis of variance. In this table,

$$B = [1/(n - 1)][N - (1/N) \sum_{i=1}^{n} T_i^2],$$

where T_i is the total number of measurements made on the ith subject $= pt_i$, and N is the total number of measurements in the study $= \sum_{i=1}^{n} T_i$. When the number of samples is the same for all subjects (t), then $B = pt$. Otherwise, B is close to the mean number of measurements per subject.

We prefer to use this formal analysis of variance only for estimating σ_b^2, and then only when the number of samples per subject is not constant. Estimating the variance components separately, starting with σ_a^2, then proceeding to σ_w^2, and finally σ_b^2, encourages inspection and testing of the data at each level of the nested analysis, particularly with respect to outliers. Moreover, the homogeneity of individual within-subject vari-

Table 6.1   Nested Analysis of Variance

Source of variance	Degrees of freedom	Expected mean squares
Among subjects	$n - 1$	$\sigma_a^2 + p\sigma_w^2 + B\sigma_b^2$
Within subjects	$(N/p) - n$	$\sigma_a^2 + p\sigma_w^2$
Between replicates within samples	$N[(p - 1)/p]$	σ_a^2
Total	$N - 1$	

ances s_i^2 should be tested before averaging them to estimate σ_w^2. Schneider believed that σ_w^2 should be the same for all subjects. If this condition does not hold, but $(\sigma_w^2)_i$ is independent of μ_i, then the formal components of variance analysis still provides an unbiased (although inefficient) estimate of among-subjects variance σ_b^2. In any case, σ_w^2 is estimated as the weighted average of s_i^2. The problem of heterogeneity of within-subject variances will reappear during this chapter and the next. Details of these analyses are set out in Section 6.4.

6.1.1 The Problem of "Run-to-Run" Analytical Variance

In the early 1960s, G. Williams and colleagues began a series of studies at the National Institutes of Health measuring 20 biochemical and 5 hematological tests in apparently healthy volunteers, drawing weekly blood specimens under fasting conditions at 8–10 A.M. for 10–12 weeks. A preliminary report by Williams appeared in 1967 and final publication of results in 1970 in three papers (Williams et al., Harris et al., and Cotlove et al.)

A chief concern of Williams and colleagues at that time was to identify "run-to-run" analytical variance resulting from variations in operating conditions from one "run" or "batch" of laboratory analyses to another. Such variations include minor changes in the composition of reagent batches or in materials used to calibrate measurement devices or in environmental conditions within the laboratory. For any biochemical analyte, ongoing quality control surveillance should reduce the total variance from such sources to a constant level. Subtracting this variance from that observed in repeated test results for a given subject would reveal the individual's biological variance.

Of course, run-to-run variations in laboratory conditions are not the only sources of analytical variance. There are also immediate causes that produce small but observable differences in replicate results from the same blood specimen (within-run variation). This component of variance may be estimated by performing all determinations in duplicate or triplicate.

Quantifying run-to-run analytical variance requires another source of data, typically the daily measurements carried out on specimens from frozen or lyophilized (condensed) serum pools or other materials used in the laboratory's quality control program. This raises the interesting question of whether the variance computed from these data is identical to the long-term analytical variance (i.e., combined within-run and run-to-run) affecting the results of patient specimens. For example, there might be interfering substances varying from time to time in a patient's serum but found only in very dilute quantities, or not at all, in the quality control material. The resulting random inaccuracy could not be accounted for by subtracting long-term variance estimated from the laboratory's quality control data. Such problems are well known to clinical chemists. One attempt to examine their practical significance was reported by Williams et al. (1977), who showed that in most, but not all analytes, routine analyses of batches of uniform control sera did provide a valid source for estimation of long-term analytical variance in patients' specimens.[2]

Some years earlier, Young et al. (1971) had published results of a study in which the run-to-run component of analytical variance was eliminated by freezing all serial specimens at $-20°C$ at the time of collection and then analyzing them during a single run at the end of the study. Comparing estimates of average within-subject variance with those found in the previous studies by Williams and coworkers (1970), a substantial decrease was noted in cholesterol and lactate dehydrogenase (LDH), a liver enzyme. Little difference was seen in other common analytes, perhaps because of the already low run-to-run analytical variance in these analytes, but probably also as a result of variability in estimates of biological variance.

---

[2] Bokelund et al. (1974) compared within-run variances from aliquots of control sera and subject specimens to isolate the effect of "preinstrumental" variables such as centrifugation and other blood-handling procedures that might inflate the variation seen in replicate determinations in patient specimens.

The idea of removing between-run analytical variance by storing serial specimens and analyzing them all in one run has proved attractive to later investigators (see below) but bears its own problems. One is the obvious constraint on the number of reference subjects that can be included in such a study design. The study of Williams et al. included 68 subjects, whereas Young et al. were able to examine only nine. Another problem is the possibility of trends showing up as a consequence of variations in the storage times of different specimens prior to analysis. These can be estimated by regression analysis, and their effects, if any, deducted from the subject's overall variance. A better solution is to avoid such trends by storing at a very low temperature such as $-80°C$.

6.2 HOMOGENEITY OF WITHIN-SUBJECT VARIANCES

The homogeneity of the biological components of within-subject variances among a group of reference subjects can be tested without separating out the analytical component if the latter is constant for all subjects. Suppose we assume that serial values of an analyte measured at least a week apart in one individual represent a sample of independent observations from a Normally distributed population of possible values in that individual during the overall time period. This is certainly more reasonable than the assumption that a cross-sectional distribution of observations is Normal. Nevertheless, it carries the underlying premise that the individual remained in a "steady state" during the sampling period and did not, for example, endure some temporary illness or medication that would systematically shift his usual level of the analyte. In practice, maintenance of a steady state requires that successive specimens be drawn at about the same time of day (to avoid circadian rhythms), that the pre-analytical condition and treatment of the subject and handling of the specimen be as uniform as possible, and, of course, that the biochemical procedure used to determine the result be the same throughout the period. Finally, laboratory practice should be well controlled so that the analytical variance remains constant. Given all of these conditions, a Normal distribution of repeated observations during a limited time period is not unreasonable!

In this case, an appropriate test for the homogeneity of within-subject variances is Bartlett's chi-square test.[3] The difficulty for our purposes with Bartlett's or any other statistical test for the homogeneity of variances is that it provides no information about the distribution of "true" within-subject variances when the hypothesis of homogeneity is rejected. However, an estimate of the variance of true variances may be obtained from the following formula (Harris, 1970):

$$\text{Var } \sigma^2_{w,i} = \{\text{Var } s_i^2 - [2/(t - 1)](\text{Mean } s_i^2)^2\}(t - 1)/(t + 1),$$

$$(6.3)$$

where $\sigma^2_{w,i}$ denotes true within-subject variance in the ith subject, s_i^2 is the observed variance, and t is the (assumed constant) number of serial values for each subject.[4] The derivation of Equation (6.3), based on the assumption that successive values measured over a limited period of time are Normally distributed, is given in Appendix 6.1.

If calculation of the right-hand side of this equation produces a negative value, then Var $\sigma^2_{w,i}$ should be assumed zero, and the homogeneity of within-subject variances accepted. Otherwise, the estimated value of Var $\sigma^2_{w,i}$ may be used in calculating a critical difference between two successive test values: the so-called reference change limit (see Chapter 7, Section 7.2.2). We turn now to a more fundamental question: What does the relative size of average within-subject to among-sub-

---

[3] As is well known, Bartlett's test, while sensitive to heterogeneity, is also sensitive to departures from a Normal distribution in the data.
[4] If the number of specimens varies slightly from person to person, the average number may be used for t. An exact formula would be obtained by substituting $2A$ and $2A + 1$ for the coefficients $(2/t - 1)$ and $(t - 1)/(t + 1)$, respectively, where A is the average value of $1/(t_i - 1)$.

jects variation tell us about the usefulness of the conventional cross-sectional reference range when applied to an individual patient?

6.3 THE RATIO OF AVERAGE WITHIN-SUBJECT TO AMONG-SUBJECTS VARIATION

A subject-specific reference range for a given analyte would be based on the mean and standard deviation of repeated, independent test values for the individual while in good health over some period of time. These statistics may be used to predict the next observation assuming continuation of this healthy state (Chapter 7, Section 7.3.2). However, the general proliferation of subject-specific reference ranges would be expensive. In practice, the upper (and lower) limits of the conventional 95 percent reference range already serve as alarms that a healthy state is being threatened. Are these cross-sectional reference limits really good enough to serve this purpose when so many studies since the pioneering work of Roger Williams have demonstrated the "biochemical individuality" of each person? More specifically, how small does the ratio of average within-subject to among-subjects standard deviations have to be before the cross-sectional reference range becomes clearly inadequate for patient monitoring?

To illustrate the situation, Figure 6.1 contrasts within-subject and among-subjects variation in serum alkaline phosphatase in healthy males vis-à-vis the group-based 95 percent reference range. This way of representing individual variability in biochemical analytes was introduced by G. Williams (1967). The methodology and units of measurement for alkaline phosphatase (King-Armstrong units) are obsolete today, but the message is clear that individual mean values may vary from one side of the reference range to the other, while within-person variability can be small in some persons and large in others. Most persons showed a range of variation well within the conventional reference range.

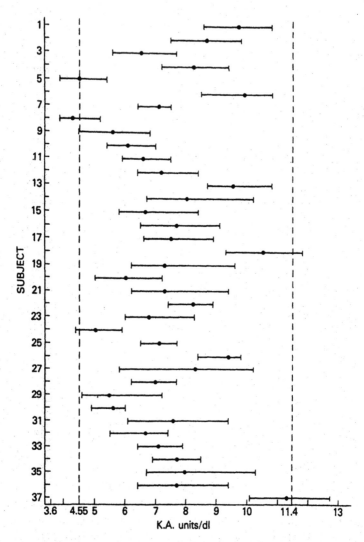

Fig. 6.1 Individual variability in alkaline phosphatase from early study of serial measurements in healthy men. (From Williams, 1967, with permission.)

We put the question in statistical terms as follows (cf. Harris, 1974). Assume that the single-sample cross-sectional distribution of observations is Normal (on original or transformed scale), and that serial testing of each reference subject would also produce a sample of observations from a Normal distribution. If μ and σ represent the mean and standard deviation of the population distribution, then the upper limit of the 95 percent reference range should be $x_U = \mu + 1.96\sigma$. Now consider the ith reference subject with true mean μ_i and standard deviation σ_i, including both biological and analytical sources of variability. For this subject, x_U is the point $\mu_i + z_i\sigma_i$, where z_i is probably greater than 1.96. Then we may write

$$\mu_i + z_i\sigma_i = \mu + 1.96\sigma$$

or

$$z_i = 1.96(\sigma/\sigma_i) + (\mu - \mu_i)/\sigma_i. \qquad (6.4)$$

The standard deviation σ represents the square root of the sum of among-subjects variance, Var μ_i, and the mean or expected value of total within-subject variance $E\sigma_i^2$. If $r = (E\sigma_i^2/\text{Var } \mu_i)^{1/2}$, and $r_i = \sigma_i/(\text{Var } \mu_i)^{1/2}$, the individual ratio, then Equation (6.4) may be rewritten as

$$z_i = 1.96[(1 + r^2)^{1/2}/r_i] - m_i/r_i, \qquad (6.5)$$

where $m_i = (\mu_i - \mu)/(\text{Var } \mu_i)^{1/2}$ is the standard Normal deviate representing the location of the ith individual's mean value in the distribution of individual means.

Suppose that the mean of the ith subject happens to be equal to the population mean μ, so that $m_i = 0$. But now suppose this individual suffers unusually high variability, say, twice the average, that is, $\sigma_i = 2 [E(\sigma_i^2)^{1/2}]$, or $r_i = 2r$. How small does the ratio r have to be for the proportion of this person's population of values outside the upper reference limit to be less than 2.5 percent? Setting the term $(1 + r^2)^{1/2}/2r$ equal to unity, we find that $r = 1/\sqrt{3} \approx 0.6$.

This implies that for any analyte characterized by a ratio of average within- to among-subjects standard deviations equal to 0.6, all individuals whose standard deviations are less than twice the average standard deviation and whose mean values over time are equal to or less than the average will find that the upper limit of the 95 percent cross-sectional reference range excludes a smaller, probably much smaller, proportion of their values than the nominal 2.5 percent. For such an analyte, and for these individuals, comparing the test value to the upper limit of the 95 percent reference range is an insensitive way of detecting an unusually high level of the analyte.

The same statement can also be made for many individuals whose mean values are greater than the average but whose within-person standard deviations are less than twice the average size. For example, if $r = 0.6$, then 70 percent of all individuals for whom $\sigma_i < 1.5 \, [E(\sigma_i^2)]^{1/2}$ will have less than 2.5 percent of their values outside the upper reference limit. This proportion rises to 87 percent of all individuals whose within-person standard deviations are less than or equal to the average standard deviation. These figures can be confirmed by setting r_i to either 0.9 or 0.6 (while $r = 0.6$) in Equation (6.5), setting $z_i = 1.96$, and solving for m_i.

One way to examine the general relationship between individual distributions of test values over time and the cross-sectional reference range is to focus on that value of m_i for which $z_i = 1.96$, in other words, that value for which the cross-sectional upper reference limit cuts off exactly 2.5 percent of the ith individual's own distribution. Let us call this value m_i^*. From Equation (6.5), m_i^* may be expressed in terms of r_i and r in the form,

$$m_i^* = 1.96[(1 + r^2)^{1/2} - r_i] \tag{6.6}$$

Figure 6.2 shows the graphs of m_i^* versus r_i/r for values of r ranging from 0.2 to 1.6. These graphs provide a great deal of information. For each value of r, any individual whose mean and standard deviation are represented by a point $(m_i, r_i/r)$ below the line for that r will find that less than 2.5 percent of

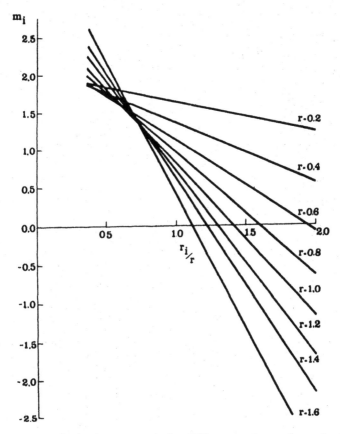

Fig. 6.2 Graphs of m_i^* versus r_i/r for different values of r, calculated from Equation (6.6). (From Harris, 1974, with permission.)

her usual values are outside the upper limit of the 95 percent reference range. For example, selecting the line corresponding to $r = 0.6$, we find, as noted earlier, that this is the case for all persons whose mean values are less than the average ($m_i < 0$) and also for a goodly proportion of those whose mean values are greater than the average ($m_i > 0$).

Conversely, any person whose mean and standard deviation are represented by a point (m_i, r_i/r) above the line for that value of r will find that more than 2.5 percent of her usual distribution of values is cut off by the upper reference limit. Can we find a value of r for which the upper reference limit is practically neutral (or should we say "equally misguided"?), that is, about half the subjects will have more and half less than 2.5 percent of their values outside the upper reference limit? At this value of r, the upper limit of the 95 percent reference range would be equally nonsensitive and nonspecific over the entire population of reference subjects. From Figure 6.2, this seems to be the case when r is about 1.4. In fact, if algebraically we equate the line segments above and below $m_i = 0$, within the bounds $r_i/r = 0.5$ to 2.0 and $m_i = -2$ to $+2$, we find that $r = 1.33$. One may interpret this for practical purposes as indicating that in the case of an analyte for which r exceeds 1.33, the cross-sectional reference limits are a reasonable basis for interpreting a test result from a patient resembling the reference subjects.

Following the publications of Williams and coworkers (1970) and Young et al. (1971), mentioned earlier, a number of studies during the next decade reported estimates of within- and among-subjects biological variation in many biochemical analytes in healthy subjects. Time spans ranged from 10 days to 5 months. Usually, only small numbers were studied (10 to 15 subjects); however, Pickup et al. (1977) monitored 37 males over 22 weeks, while Williams et al. (1978) examined 1105 men and women in young adult, middle, and older age groups as part of an ongoing health screening and maintenance program. The values used to estimate biological variation were obtained during a 5–12 week baseline period. Their results showed only narrow differences among the age–gender groups with respect to the ratio of average within- to among-subjects standard deviations, except for creatine kinase, where younger women showed substantially higher within-subject and lower among-subjects variation than older women. Other studies included those of Statland et al. (1976), Van Steirteghem et al.(1978), and Raun et al. (1982). In the studies of Pickup et al., Statland et al., and Van Steirteghem et al., specimens were deep frozen after collection and analyzed in random order shortly after the end of the collection period to eliminate the effects of between-run analytical variation. The latter was estimated from quality control samples during the course of the study.

6.3.1 Summary of Ratios

In 1982, Ross published a valuable review and summary of this work to date. Finding that the estimates of within-subject biological CV (coefficient of variation) for any analyte did not increase with increasing time span (from 10 days to 22 weeks), Ross averaged these estimates. He then associated the average for each analyte with corresponding values of long-term and short-term (within-run) analytical CV's at concentrations within the 95 percent reference range. These were taken from contemporary U.S.-wide quality proficiency evaluation programs (Ross et al., 1980) and represented the current state of the art in laboratory performance. This enabled comparison of total within-subject and among-subjects standard deviations for each analyte through the ratio r.

Table 6.2 presents results for many common and not-so-common analytes taken from Ross's summary and for specialized serum proteins from the data reported by Statland et al. (1976). The analytes are divided into separate sections for the following subranges of r values: <0.6, 0.6–<1.0, 1.0–<1.4, and ≥1.4.

One can see from this table that in many analytes analytical variation was a substantial contributor to total within-subject variation. In the decade and more since Ross's review, the analytical state of the art has improved, and many of these r values might now be considerably less than appears here. Further, it is likely that an increasing number of highly specific proteins will be determined in clinical laboratories, driven by disease-related research in molecular biology and genetics. Such analytes will undoubtedly show high degrees of individuality as evidenced by small values of r.

Table 6.2 Analytical and Biological CV's and Ratios (r) of Average Within-Subject to Among-Subjects Standard Deviations

Analyte	Analytical[a]	Within-subject biological	Among-subjects	r[b]
$r < 0.6$				
Haptoglobulin	3.1	8.8	70.5	0.13
Orosomusicoid	5.4	11.1	43.1	0.29
Transferrin	3.8	2.5	9.5	0.48
α_1-Antitrypsin	4.1	2.9	15.7	0.32
α_2-Macroglobulin	2.9	3.1	16.6	0.26
Immunoglobulin G	2.9	2.7	18.1	0.22
Immunoglobulin A	4.6	3.5	41.1	0.14
Immunoglobulin M	5.3	3.1	54.0	0.11
Complement C3	5.5	3.8	19.7	0.34
Complement C4	5.6	5.9	35.6	0.23
Alkaline phosphatase	6.3	6.3	25.3	0.25
Cholesterol	3.9	5.4	15.4	0.43
Triglyceride	5.3	27.0	58.0	0.47
$0.6 \leq r < 1.0$				
Uric acid	2.8	7.8	13.4	0.62
Lactate dehydrogenase	6.3	7.2	14.4	0.66
Bilirubin	9.2	25.0	35.2	0.76
Creatinine	6.8	4.6	10.6	0.77
Urea nitrogen	4.5	13.0	16.9	0.81
Phosphorus	3.0	7.8	9.4	0.89
Aspartate transaminase	8.7	16.0	19.7	0.92
Creatinine kinase	12.0	56.0	60.5	0.95
$1.0 \leq r < 1.4$				
Total protein	2.3	2.7	3.7	0.96
Glucose	3.4	6.2	6.4	1.1
Calcium	2.2	1.4	2.2	1.2
Iron	4.6	27.0	23.4	1.2
Potassium	1.9	5.1	4.4	1.2
Albumin	3.0	3.1	3.3	1.3
Thyroxine	7.7	8.8	8.8	1.3

Table 6.2 Continued

Analyte	Analytical[a]	Within-subject biological	Among-subjects	r[b]
$1.4 \leq r$				
Chloride	1.6	1.7	1.4	1.7
Sodium	1.1	0.74	0.60	2.2

[a] Analytical CV represents the estimate of combined run-to-run and within-run CV given by the respective sources.

[b] r is computed as the ratio of total within-subject CV to among-subjects CV, where within-subject CV is the square root of the sum of squares of analytical CV and biological within-subject CV.

Source: Data for the first 10 analytes were taken from Statland et al. (1976), Tables 1 and 2; data for the remaining 20 analytes were taken from Ross (1982, Tables 7 and 8).

Fraser (1988) has provided an exhaustive listing of estimates of biological variation (CV) in many analytes, both within and among healthy subjects, in serum and urine, that have appeared in the literature since Ross's review. In addition, a number of studies during this period estimated average within-subject biological variation in patients with various pathologies, and Fraser has listed these separately. In most of these studies, the between-run component of analytical variation was eliminated by maintaining samples at very low temperatures until the end of the collection period when they were analyzed in random order within a single run. This maneuver has the advantage of providing an unencumbered estimate of within-subject biological variation (after deducting within-run analytical variance), especially useful in the development of goals for analytical precision (see Chapter 8). However, monitoring the biochemical status of real patients necessarily involves both between- and within-run analytical variation together with biologically induced changes. Therefore, reference values used in patient management must account directly or implicitly for the contribution of long-term analytical variability. This problem reappears in Chapter 7.

6.4 EXAMPLE

When statistical tests for outliers were discussed in Chapter 3, we were primarily concerned with the distribution of the collective of observations and whether an outlying observation was a member of the same distribution as its fellows, assuming that it was not simply the result of a blunder in the biochemical determination or in record-keeping. At this point, however, our primary concern about outliers is with their effects on estimates of the variance components, σ_a^2, σ_w^2, and σ_b^2. Squared functions of the data, like variances, are highly sensitive to outliers. Since the estimates of the first two of these components are averages of observed within-specimen and within-subject variances, we want to be sure that any lack of homogeneity among these variances is not due to the effects of one or a few aberrant observations on the variances they contribute to. Therefore, the statistical methods are chosen to examine the effects of outliers on the homogeneity of variances rather than the homogeneity of the original data, although, of course, an aberrant value may affect both.

The data examined here are serial measurements of immunoglobulin G (IgG) from a recent study by Ford et al. (1988) of 12 healthy volunteers, six men and six women, ages 23–48. Altogether, 111 specimens were collected at intervals of 1 to 3 weeks, between 8:00 and 9:30 A.M.: ten specimens from seven subjects, nine from two subjects, eight from two subjects, and seven from one subject. All specimens were stored at $-30°C$ and assayed in one run by a single analyst. Each serum specimen was analyzed in duplicate. The statistical analysis described below is adapted from Fraser and Harris (1989).

6.4.1 Variance of Replicate Determinations

We start with the variance of replicate determinations on the same specimen. Assume that the deviations of a set of replicate measurements from their mean value are mutually independent and represent a random sample from a Normal population of deviations. Then, the variable $(p - 1)s_j^2/\sigma_a^2$, where s_j^2 is the variance of the p replicate determinations on the jth specimen, is distributed in a chi-square distribution with $(p - 1)$ degrees of freedom (χ_{p-1}^2). In this example, $p = 2$, so the distribution of s_j^2 should be χ_1^2 multiplied by σ_a^2. Percentiles of χ_1^2 are listed in Table 6.3.

A complete listing of the IgG measurements obtained by Ford et al. is given in Appendix 6.1, by subject and duplicates within each specimen. The cumulative distribution of the variances of duplicates is plotted in Figure 6.3. The true variance σ_a^2 may be estimated by the mean value, 165.59 (mg/dL)^2. Multiplying the percentiles in Table 6.3 by this value, we obtain the expected cumulative distribution of the variances, plotted as a smooth curve in Figure 6.3. The fit is fine between the 60th and

Table 6.3 Percentiles of the Chi-Square Distribution with One Degree of Freedom (χ_1^2)

Percentile	χ_1^2
2.5	0.000982
5.0	0.00393
10.0	0.0158
20.0	0.0642
30.0	0.148
40.0	0.275
50.0	0.455
60.0	0.708
70.0	1.074
80.0	1.642
90.0	2.706
95.0	3.841
97.5	5.024
99.0	6.635
99.9	7.879

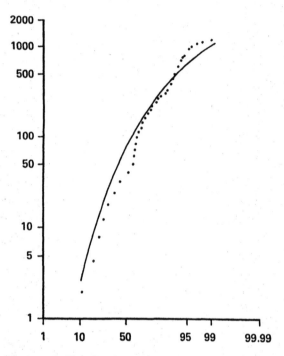

Fig. 6.3 Observed distribution of variances of duplicates. Smooth curve represents expected distribution if all observed values were estimates of a common true variance (From Fraser and Harris, 1989. Reprinted by permission of CRC Press, Boca Raton, Florida.)

90th percentiles of the distribution, but up to the 60th percentile, the observed variances are smaller than expected, given the mean value, while beyond the 90th percentile, the variances are larger than expected.

Suppose we experiment with the goodness of fit by deleting the 11 variances greater than 500 $(mg/dL)^2$. This lowers the mean to 90.24 $(mg/dL)^2$. Using this as the estimate of σ_a^2, and fitting the χ_1^2 distribution to the remaining 100 variances shows excellent fit up to about the 70th percentile of the reduced set; however, above this point, variances are again larger than expected. Since duplicates from all the specimens were analyzed in random order, there is no reason for thinking that very small variances might indicate some nonrandom bias favoring nearly identical duplicate results. Therefore, there is no basis for further experimenting by deleting a group of small variances.

The mean value of the 22 determinations that yielded unexpectedly large variances between duplicates was very little different from the mean of all the data. Without more information about details of the biochemical analysis, we are left with chance alone to explain the upper 10 percent of duplicate variances. However, since no one or two pairs of duplicates showed exceptionally large variances, the average duplicate variance, 165.59 $(mg/dL)^2$ may be accepted as the best estimate s_a^2 of within-run analytical variance.

Before leaving the assessment of variation between duplicates, we might ask how large an extreme variance should be before we reject it as an outlier significantly larger than the remaining values. To help answer this question, we test the ratio of the maximum variance to the sum of all variances (Cochran, 1941). Critical values for this ratio at the 0.05 and 0.01 levels of significance are tabulated in Dixon and Massey (1983, Table A-17). They depend on the number of variances and the degrees of freedom for each, assumed constant. For one degree of freedom per variance and 120 variances (as close as the table comes to 111), the critical values of the ratio are 0.1 at the 5 percent level and 0.12 at the 1 percent level. The sum of all the observed variances between duplicates is 18,380.5, so that a new, extreme value would have to exceed the value x, where $x/(18,380.5 + x) = 0.1$, or 2,042, to be significant at the 5 percent level. This is 70 percent larger than the largest observed variance.

6.4.2   Within-Subject Variances

Cochran's test may also be applied to the extreme value observed among a set of within-subject variances. Each such variance should be calculated as the variance of the means of replicate determinations for that subject. It is possible that the variances of replicates conform well to expectations, but the mean(s) of one or two replicate measurements are so different from those obtained for the other specimens that the within-subject variance is greatly inflated. This might be the result of undetected contamination of that specimen, or an interfering substance in the subject's serum at the time of sampling, or some temporary biasing factor in the biochemical analysis.

Table 6.4 lists the within-subject variances observed for the 12 subjects in the study of Ford et al. (1988). The ratio of the maximum to the sum of the variances is 3134.65/21085.16 = 0.15. The average number of specimens is 9.25. Critical values of Cochran's test for 12 variances and six to nine degrees of freedom range from 0.21 to 0.24 at the 5 percent level of significance. Clearly, none of these variances is a significant outlier.

Weighting each of these within-subject variances by its degrees of freedom (number of specimens minus 1), their mean and variance come to 1755.33 and 525,416.96, respectively. Ap-

Table 6.4 Variances of Means of Duplicate Values of IgG in 12 Subjects

Subject	Number of specimens	Variance (mg/dL)^2
1	10	3134.65
2	10	1910.51
3	10	2612.07
4	9	1614.69
5	10	388.84
6	9	1956.09
7	10	1598.89
8	8	1246.58
9	10	950.56
10	8	2243.25
11	7	1812.71
12	10	1616.32
Totals	111	21085.16

Source: Fraser and Harris (1989, Table A2). Reprinted by permission of CRC Press, Boca Raton, Florida.

plying Equation (6.3) with $t = 9.25$, a strongly negative result is obtained for Var $\sigma_{w,i}^2$, indicating that σ_w^2 is constant for all subjects. Its estimated value is $s_w^2 = $ mean $s_i^2 - (s_a^2)/p = 1755.33 - (165.59/2) = 1672.53$ (mg/dL)^2, or $s_w = 40.90$ mg/dL.

6.4.3 Among-Subjects Variance

Before estimating this component of variance, we should examine the distribution of mean values for any possibly significant outliers. These means are listed in Table 6.5. Our hypothesis is that these means are a random sample from a homogeneous Normal distribution. To test whether an outlying mean represents a subject from a different population than the others, we suggest the Dixon ratio D/R, cited in Chapter 3, Section 3.4, where D is the difference between the extreme value and its nearest neighbor and R is the range of all the means. Critical

Table 6.5 Mean IgG
Concentrations in 12 Subjects

Subject	Mean (mg/dL)
1	1010.0
2	803.2
3	905.2
4	952.2
5	666.2
6	1019.9
7	945.8
8	971.6
9	1107.1
10	1080.3
11	915.9
12	903.0

Source: Fraser and Harris (1989, Table A3).
Reprinted by permission of CRC Press,
Boca Raton, Florida.

values at the 5 percent and 1 percent levels of significance for sample sizes up to 30 are given by Barnett and Lewis (1994, Table XIXa). For sample size 12, the critical value at $P = 0.05$ is 0.376. From Table 6.5, the ratio D/R is $(803.2 - 666.2)/(1107.1 - 666.2) = 0.31$. We have no reason to reject the hypothesis that all subject means come from the same population.

To this point, then, the data have been tested for homogeneity of variances of duplicate determinations, homogeneity of within-subject variances, and the significance of outliers among subject variances and mean values. In the process, two variance components have been estimated: (within-run) analytical variance σ_a^2 and average within-subject variance σ_w^2. The latter is purely biological in this case because run-to-run analytical variance has been eliminated in the design of the study.

The remaining component, among-subjects variance σ_b^2, may now be estimated according to the analysis of variance given in Table 6.1. This requires calculating the quantity B because the number of specimens collected was not the same for all subjects (Table 6.4). As noted earlier, B is approximately equal to the average number of measurements per subject, in this case, the number of replicates per specimen times the average number of specimens per subject: 2(9.25), or 18.50. More precisely,

$$B = [(1/(n - 1))][N - (1/N) \sum_{i=1}^{n} T_i^2]$$

$$= (1/11)[222 - (1/222)(4156)] = 18.48.$$

Carrying through the analysis of variance produced the results shown in Table 6.6. Following the mean square formulas in Table 6.1, the estimate of σ_w^2 is computed as $(3510.64 - 165.59)/2$, or 1672.53, in agreement with the value obtained earlier from the weighted average of within-subject variances. The estimated value of σ_b^2 is $s_b^2 = (276{,}079.4 - 3510.64)/18.48 = 14{,}749.39$, or $s_b = 121.45$ mg/dL.

Table 6.6 Nested Analysis of Variance for IgG Data
($n = 12$, $N = 222$)

Source of variation	Degrees of freedom	Mean square
Among subjects	11	276,079.4
Within subject	99	3,510.64
Between duplicates	111	165.59

Source: Fraser and Harris (1989, Table A5). Reprinted by permission of CRC Press, Boca Raton, Florida.

When both the number of specimens per subject and the number of replicates per specimen are constant, a formal analysis of variance may be dispensed with entirely. In this case,

$$s_b^2 = [(ntp - 1)/tp(n - 1)]$$
$$\times [s_T^2 - s_a^2 - (N - 2)/(N - 1)(s_w^2)], \quad (6.6)$$

where s_T^2 is the variance of all N determinations. For the IgG data, $s_T^2 = 15,397.32$ (mg/dL)^2. Using this formula with $t = 9.25$ and the estimates s_a^2 and s_w^2 given above, $s_b = 121.38$, very close to the ANOVA estimate even though the number of specimens per subject varied somewhat.

To determine the ratio $r = (Es_i^2/\widehat{\text{Var}}\,\mu_i)^{1/2}$ for IgG, an estimate of analytical variance including both between- and within-run components needs to be added to s_w^2. Statland et al. (1976), cited earlier, list the CV of the run-to-run component for IgG at 2.4 percent and the within-run CV at 1.6 percent. The latter figure is close to the corresponding CV of 1.4 percent in the data here [$100(165.59)^{1/2}/936.76$], where 936.76 is the weighted mean of the subject means given in Table 6.5. Total analytical CV is estimated at [$(2.4)^2 + (1.6)^2]^{1/2} = 2.9$ percent, or 27.2 mg/dL. Combining this with s_w yields an estimate of $(Es_i^2)^{1/2}$ equal to [$(27.2)^2 + (40.9)^2]^{1/2}$, or 49.1 mg/dL. Then $r = 49.1/121.45 = 0.4$. This is almost twice the value of r given for IgG in Table 6.2, because the CV of within-subject biological variation [$100(40.9/$

936.76)], or 4.4 percent, is higher than that found by Statland et al., while the CV for among-subjects variation [100(121.45/936.76)], or 13.0 percent, is lower (see Table 6.2). Nevertheless, r remains considerably less than 0.6, confirming the need for a subject-specific reference range to properly interpret an individual's test result for this analyte.

**APPENDIX 6.1   ESTIMATING VARIANCE OF TRUE
                 WITHIN-SUBJECT VARIANCES**

To derive Equation (6.3) relating Var $\sigma^2_{w,i}$, Var s_i^2, and mean s_i^2, where $\sigma^2_{w,i}$ is the "true" within-subject variance of the ith subject and s_i^2 is the observed variance based on the results of t serial determinations:

For convenience, we will omit the subscripts on σ^2 and s^2. Assuming the results are mutually independent and a random sample from a Normal distribution, the conditional distribution of s^2, given σ^2, is a gamma distribution,

$$\Gamma(s^2 \mid \sigma^2) = (k/2\sigma^2)^{k/2}[(s^2)^{(k-2)/2}/\Gamma(k/2)] \exp(-ks^2/2\sigma^2),$$

where $k = t - 1$. Then, the mean and variance are $E(s^2 \mid \sigma^2) = \sigma^2$, and Var$(s^2 \mid \sigma^2) = 2\sigma^4/k$.

If $f(s^2)$ denotes the unconditional distribution of s^2; and $g(\sigma^2)$, the distribution of σ^2, then

$$f(s^2) = \int_0^\infty \Gamma(s^2 \mid \sigma^2)g(\sigma^2)\,d\sigma^2.$$

Thus, $f(s^2)$ can be thought of as the weighted average distribution of $s^2 \mid \sigma^2$ with the probabilities of different values of σ^2 as the weights. An important formula in the theory of conditional distributions relates the unconditional variance of a variable Y to its conditional variance and mean with respect to another variable X; that is,

$$\text{Var } Y = E[\text{Var}(Y \mid X)] + \text{Var}[E(Y \mid X)].$$

Here $Y = s^2$ and $X = \sigma^2$. The first term on the right-hand side is $2(E\sigma^4)/k = (2/k)[\text{Var } \sigma^2 + (E\sigma^2)^2]$, and the second term is Var σ^2. Therefore,

$$\text{Var } s^2 = (\text{Var } \sigma^2)[(k + 2)/k] + (E\sigma^2)^2 (2/k).$$

Then, estimating $E\sigma^2$ as mean s^2,

$$\text{Estimated Var}(\sigma^2) = [\text{Var } s^2 - (2/k)(\text{mean } s^2)^2][k/(k + 2)],$$

which is Equation (6.3) in the text.

APPENDIX 6.2 DATA SETS: SERIAL MEASUREMENTS OF IMMUNOGLOBULIN G (IgG)

Subject	Duplicate determinations in each specimen		
1	1006	989	1033
	1016	988	1048
	1014	996	1086
	1032	1003	1081
	997	872	991
	1016	888	997
	1075		
	1071		

Subject	Duplicate determinations in each specimen		
2	803	809	788
	801	803	797
	896	827	788
	887	818	779
	714	823	804
	715	830	792
	792		
	797		
3	860	808	944
	868	799	951
	967	922	906
	963	918	913
	856	920	960
	850	910	959
	914		
	916		

Subject	Duplicate determinations in each specimen		
4	999	957	874
	1007	966	923
	987	925	893
	990	929	890
	988	925	978
	987	955	963
5	680	651	697
	677	652	707
	665	669	670
	667	669	664
	638	675	681
	641	672	677
	617		
	655		

Subject	Duplicate determinations in each specimen		
6	1044	1067	1031
	1027	1043	1054
	1017	1049	1036
	1009	1024	1022
	910	1019	1055
	910	994	1048
7	958	942	947
	950	964	950
	963	910	950
	979	916	941
	934	883	1050
	927	890	1022
	932		
	908		
8	970	945	981
	959	993	973

Subject	Duplicate determinations in each specimen		
	953	912	972
	952	922	946
	997	1030	
	992	1049	
9	1123	1171	1058
	1105	1136	1069
	1104	1072	1108
	1095	1069	1080
	1118	1125	1100
	1096	1115	1084
	1168		
	1146		
10	996	1133	1073
	1036	1089	1064
	1111	1005	1091
	1119	1010	1113

Subject	Duplicate determinations in each specimen		
	1067	1127	
	1099	1152	
11	874	949	904
	871	950	907
	944	834	980
	920	873	971
	933		
	913		
12	857	823	925
	902	808	972
	946	918	924
	925	950	902
	853	922	930
	872	902	917
	896		
	916		

Data available through the courtesy of C. G. Fraser, Department of Biochemical Medicine, Ninewells Hospital and Medical School, Dundee, Scotland.

7

PREDICTIVE VALUES FOR MONITORING HEALTHY SUBJECTS AND PATIENTS

7.1   INTRODUCTION

In this chapter, we describe various statistical methods for monitoring healthy subjects or outpatients after treatment. In the first case—monitoring healthy subjects—within-subject variances play the central role. Observations are generally scheduled at long intervals (at least every 6 months, often annually or even less frequently), and deviations from the appointed times are relatively minor. The immediate problem is that of judging the significance of a change between the initial measurement of an analyte and the next observation. To resolve this we must use information about within-subject variances obtained from repeated measurements in other healthy subjects. When several serial measurements of the analyte become available while the individual remains in a steady state, we can turn to methods of deriving predictive ranges that rely solely on the person's own past record. Such methods, and the statistical models behind them, are necessarily relatively simple.

In monitoring patients, the prediction problem is more difficult. Not only are lengths of series short, but, more importantly, the scheduled interval between measurements is also usually relatively short. In outpatients, for example, a 3-month interval is commonly recommended. In practice, observations often occur at irregular times, and this variation is not negligible relative to the scheduled interval. In this situation, developing reference values for monitoring observations in a new patient requires results obtained from multiple series in previous patients. Recent work in this area appears very promising, but the mathematical structure involved is complex.

To start, we examine methods familiar to many clinical laboratory workers for obtaining a reference criterion to judge the atypicality of a change between the initial test value and the next one.[1] Such a criterion has been called a *reference change*

---

[1] We are concerned here with a simple difference between two successive observations while the subject is in the same biochemical state. We are not referring to a *conditional* change from a given (i.e., fixed)

value (Harris and Brown, 1979; Harris and Yasaka, 1983; Boyd and Harris, 1986) or a *critical difference* (e.g., Costongs et al., 1985). Most recently, Kairisto et al. (1993) have suggested *reference change limit* in analogy to the limit of a cross-sectional reference range. Although reference change value or limit may be a slightly more awkward-sounding expression than critical difference, it is a reminder that we are still talking about reference values in laboratory medicine. Before any of these terms became current, however, clinical laboratories were familiar with another name, the *delta check*, used to help solve a related problem in quality control. For background and later comparison, our discussion begins with a review of the delta check.

7.2 COMPARISON OF TWO SERIAL RESULTS

7.2.1 The Delta Check

The idea of comparing the current test value of a patient with the previous one is well known in the clinical laboratory, where the difference between the two results is commonly called a *delta*, and the comparison with a designated critical difference is called a *delta check*. The name was originally proposed by Nosanchuk and Gottmann (1974). The same idea was also suggested, apparently independently, by Whitehurst et al. (1975) and was further recommended by Ladenson (1975) and Sher (1979). These authors saw the delta check as a way of taking advantage of computerized cumulative reporting systems then being introduced into clinical laboratory computing systems. The primary objective was to detect a possible misidentification of a patient specimen or some mistake in the analytical procedure. In this case, the error would be corrected by reanalyzing the current specimen or obtaining a new one. Otherwise, the current result would be confirmed and reported to the clinician with the notation that it had been rechecked and confirmed.

---

initial value. Conditional changes were discussed in Chapter 5 in the context of time-dependent reference limits.

In the original studies of delta checking, the delta variable was either the absolute difference between current and previous test values or the percentage change of current value from the earlier result. For example, Whitehurst et al. used the absolute difference when the previous value was within the "normal range," the percentage change when that value was above the normal range. The critical difference (or percentage) for any analyte was chosen subjectively but guided by estimates of analytical variation derived from quality control data. Ladenson noted that at first, he tried to use the (average) within-subject biological variation reported by Young et al. (1971), but found that this produced "an unmanageable number" of discrepancies between current and previous values.

In a series of reports, Wheeler and Sheiner (1977), Sheiner et al. (1979a), and Wheeler and Sheiner (1981) examined the frequency distribution of observed differences between consecutive results of electrolytes, creatinine, and urea nitrogen measured in patient specimens through a multichannel analyzer. They selected specimen pairs in which the time interval between results was 0.9–2.5 days and chose as critical differences the 5th and 95th percentiles of the distribution for each analyte. The delta check criteria of Whitehurst and Ladenson were also applied. In addition, the authors explored differences in urea nitrogen/creatinine ratios and in anion gaps (electrolyte balance), medically important combinations of these analytes.

They found, as had earlier investigators, that most of the differences outside the chosen bounds were not attributable to some type of laboratory mishandling of the specimen, but were confirmed valid results, sometimes but usually not explainable by reference to patients' written records. These apparently "false-positive" discrepancies were believed due to effects of intervening therapy or disease processes not unexpected in an acute care hospital. Thus, Wheeler and Sheiner (1981) concluded that "with the delta check methods one can detect (laboratory) errors otherwise overlooked, but at the cost of investigating many false positives. . . ."

Lacher and Connelly (1988) reported percentiles of the distribution of differences between current and previous results for 12 serum chemistry tests in the University of Minnesota clinical laboratories. They also tabulated percentiles of *rate checks*, defined as the difference divided by the time interval between samples. In more than 50 percent of pairs, this interval was less than 2.5 days. For one analyte, creatinine, Lacher and Connelly compared the 2.5th and 97.5th percentiles of the deltas from ten different wards of the hospital, including, for example, general pediatrics, two surgical/medical wards, the surgical intensive care unit, and the dialysis ward. As would be expected, substantial differences appeared among these wards at both the very low (negative) and very high (positive) percentiles of the delta values.

None of the earlier papers on delta checking had presented separate distributions (or percentiles) of delta values for the different wards from which patients' specimens originated. All based their critical differences for each analyte on the combined distribution of deltas between current and previous determinations within a given time interval. Establishing separate criteria for different services or groups of services would undoubtedly reduce the heterogeneity of observed deltas (Boyd and Harris, 1986, discussed later). If further investigation of delta checks along these lines enhances their ability to detect medically important discrepancies, this function of the delta check may prove as valuable to the clinical laboratory as revealing the rare occurrence of a mixup in specimen identification or some other laboratory blunder. At present, most clinical laboratorians regard delta checking as an internal, potentially powerful device to help laboratory personnel recognize and correct serious unpredictable mistakes in operations before the erroneous reports leave the laboratory. The method is nonparametric and empirical but limited to dealing with just two observations from each patient.

One practical advantage of deriving delta check criteria directly from a distribution of observed differences between two test results is that the analyst does not have to deal explicitly with possible heterogeneity in within-patient variances or a correlation between the test values. A nonzero correlation is not unlikely when the time interval between specimens is only 1 or 2 days. Heterogeneity of variances would increase the variance of differences, whereas positive correlation would decrease the variance, but, in any case, their net effect has already been built into the empirical distribution. This imposes a subtle restriction, however: the analyst is not free to choose a specific level of within-patient variance to use in constructing the delta check acceptance criterion. The reference change method presented below removes this restriction.

Healthy subjects in a health maintenance program provide only infrequent specimens for biochemical analysis. To develop a criterion for comparing the first two observations in such cases, we turn to a more formal statistical method, looking toward the calculation of subject-specific predictive ranges when a series of observations are available.

7.2.2 Reference Change Limits

Reference change limits may be derived from a general time series model, the first-order autoregressive model, defined later for monitoring patients over extended periods of time. At this stage, since only two observations are involved, no explicit time series model is necessary but only elementary statistical formulas. If $x_i(t_1)$ and $x_i(t_2)$ (or x_{i1} and x_{i2}, for short) represent determinations at times t_1 and t_2 in the ith subject, and d_i is the difference between them, then

$$\text{Variance}(d_i) = \sigma_i^2(x_{i,1}) + \sigma_i^2(x_{i,2}) - 2R_i(1,2) \qquad (7.1)$$

where the σ_i^2's are the variances of the respective observations, and R_i is their correlation.[2] Assuming the variance (including both analytical and biological components) is constant for both

---

[2] We use R here rather than the more usual symbol ρ to denote correlation because ρ will be used in the first-order autoregressive model to represent the correlation between the actual (circulating) levels of the analyte being measured, not the determinations that include errors of measurement.

observations, this formula reduces to

$$\text{Variance}(d_i) = 2\sigma_i^2(1 - R_i). \tag{7.2}$$

The subscript i indicates that both within-subject variance and the correlation between two successive results may be specific to the ith individual. However, when measurements are separated by long intervals of time, R_i is usually assumed equal to zero. Further, since only one observation precedes the current measurement, information about σ_i^2 must be obtained from sources outside the ith individual—for example, from serial measurements in similar persons or from average variances reported in the literature (e.g., Chapter 6, Table 6.2).

The reference change limit is therefore a group-based index like the conventional "upper limit of normal," but based on variances. The question then arises: Should we use the average variance or examine the homogeneity of within-subject variances? If these variances appear to be heterogeneous among individuals similar to the person under study, then, from Equation (6.3) and information about the distribution of observed variances, we may be able to reconstruct the underlying distribution of true variances σ_i^2. This would allow selection of a higher percentile of this distribution than that represented by the average value, reducing the probability of a false-positive difference. This has been the general approach taken in the original papers on reference change limits (Harris and Brown, 1979; Harris and Yasaka, 1983) and, more recently, by Boyd and Harris (1986), Caudill and Boone (1986), and Queraltó et al. (1993).

It has been our experience that in the great majority of analytes, observed within-subject variances s_i^2 follow approximately logNormal distributions although outliers often appear. Examples from Queraltó et al. (1993) are shown in Figure 7.1.

Robust estimates of the mean and variance of $\log_e s_i^2$ may be obtained through Healy's trimming procedure (1979).[3] These

---

[3] This procedure somewhat overestimates the true variance and should be applied only when outliers appear in the observed sample.

estimates are then converted to the mean and variance of s_i^2 using standard formulas relating the mean and variance of a logNormally distributed variable to the mean and variance of its logarithm, as follows:

$$\text{Mean } s_i^2 = \exp[\text{Mean log } s_i^2 + (\text{Var log } s_i^2)/2]$$

$$\text{Var } s_i^2 = (\text{Mean } s_i^2)^2[\exp(\text{Var log } s_i^2) - 1].$$

(7.3)

Then, using Equation (6.3), an estimate of the standard deviation of true variances σ_i^2 may be obtained. The estimate of Mean σ_i^2 is the mean of s_i^2. A logNormal distribution of s_i^2 implies that σ_i^2 is also distributed in logNormal form (Harris, 1970). Therefore, using Equations (7.3) in terms of σ_i^2 to solve for the mean and variance of log σ_i^2, percentiles of σ_i^2 may be estimated from tables of the Normal distribution. A BASIC program to execute these steps is given in Appendix 7.1.

Now, let D_p be a difference such that $|D_p|/1.96$ is a specified percentile p of the standard deviation of d_i. That is, assuming $R_i = 0$ in Equation (7.2), $D_p^2 = 2(1.96)^2\sigma_p^2$, where σ_p^2 is the estimated pth percentile of the distribution of σ_i^2. Plotting $|D_p|$ on probability paper, we obtain a graph of the estimated proportion of individuals in whom a change of $|D_p|$ units between the current and previous result would be statistically significant at the 0.05 level of probability. The selected value of $|D_p|$ becomes the reference change limit. Of course, the clinical sensitivity and specificity of the reference change limit can only be determined by experience.

Figure 7.2 presents graphs of possible reference change limits $|D_p|$ for serum calcium in each sex (Harris and Yasaka, 1983). This study included 286 women and 412 men enrolled in health screening programs in Osaka and Tokyo. Each individual had undergone 15–18 semiannual screening examinations.

Figure 7.2 indicates, for example, that a change of 0.20 mmol/L between two consecutive observations would be statistically significant at the 0.05 level in about 40 percent of women and 50 percent of men. However, a change of 0.25 mmol/L

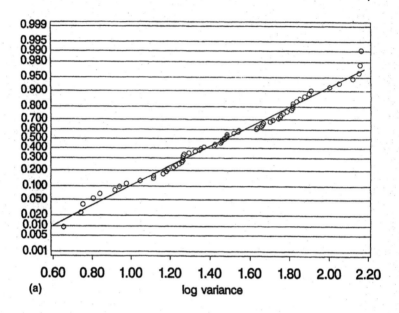

(a)   log variance

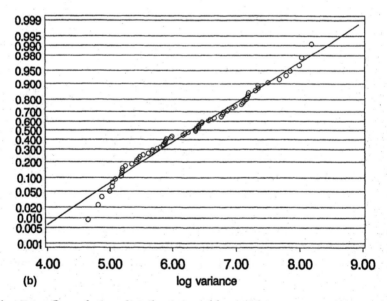

(b)   log variance

Fig. 7.1 Cumulative distributions of log within-person variance for four analytes: (a) albumin, (b) alkaline phosphatase, (c) cholesterol, (d) potassium. (From Queraltó et al., 1993, with permission.)

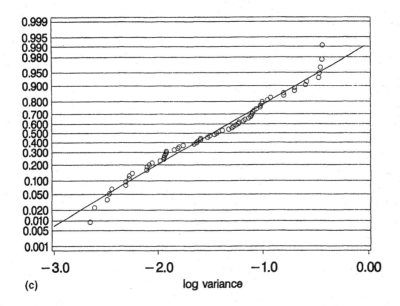

(c)

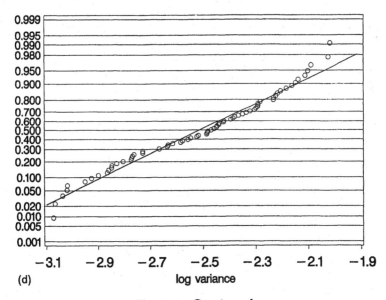

(d)

Fig. 7.1 Continued.

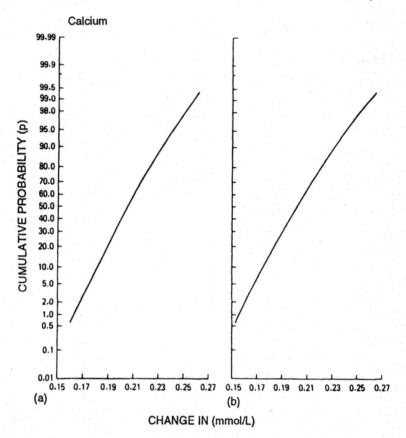

Fig. 7.2 Expected proportion of individuals in whom a specified change $|D_p|$ in two calcium measurements 6 months apart would be statistically significant at the 5 percent probability level, by sex: (a) women, (b) men. (From Harris and Yasaka, 1983, with permission.)

would be significant in about 95 percent of persons of either sex.

7.2.3 Comparison of Delta Check and Reference Change Limits

In a study permitting direct comparison between delta checking as typically performed in a clinical laboratory and reference change limits, Boyd and Harris (1986) reviewed patient data

Table 7.1   Average Correlation Coefficients at One-Day Intervals[a]

Test	Surgical intensive care (51 patients)	Orthopedic surgery (51 patients)	Obstetrics/ gynecology (21 patients)
Urea nitrogen	0.58	0.56	0.31
Sodium	0.35	0.23	0.07
Potassium	0.12	0.35	−0.08
Chloride	0.37	0.22	−0.11
Carbon dioxide	0.27	0.12	−0.22
Glucose	0.09	0.07	0.09
Creatinine	0.53	0.05	0.16

[a] Under the hypothesis that within-patient correlation coefficients are homogeneous with a true mean of zero, individual estimates will be approximately Normal with standard deviation equal to $1/n^{1/2}$, where n is the number of serial observations (Box and Jenkins, 1970, p. 35). Given $n \geq 4$, then under this hypothesis, the standard error of a mean correlation would be ≤ 0.07 for results from the surgical intensive care and othopedic surgery units and ≤ 0.11 for results from the obstetrics/gynecology unit.
Source: Boyd and Harris (1986), p. 119.

from three different services (nursing units) at the University of Virginia Hospital: an orthopedic surgery ward, a surgical intensive care unit, and an obstetrics/gynecology ward. The time interval between analyses was fixed at 1 day. All patients who had at least four successive results were included in the subsequent determination of reference change limits. The seven most commonly requested analytes were studied: sodium, potassium, chloride, carbon dioxide, glucose, urea nitrogen and creatinine. Estimates of the average correlation between consecutive observations varied considerably among analytes and among the different services as may be seen in Table 7.1.

These average correlations ($\bar{r}$) were substituted for R_i in Equation (7.2) and reference change limits calculated as $|D_p| = [2(1.96)^2 \sigma_p^2 (1 - \bar{r})]^{1/2}$.[4] Figure 7.3 shows the graphs of $|D_p|$ for

---

[4] Within-subject correlations, like within-subject variances, should be tested for homogeneity, or at least for outliers, before averaging. As-

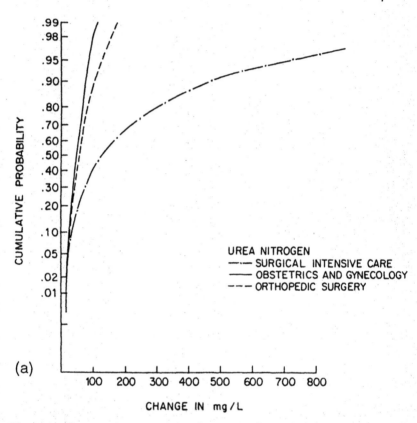

Fig. 7.3 Expected proportion of patients from different hospital services in whom a specified daily change in urea nitrogen (a) or sodium (b) would be statistically significant at the 5 percent probability level. (From Boyd and Harris, 1986, reprinted by permission of S. Karger AG, Basel.)

suming true mean different from zero, the well-known z-transform may be used to normalize the distribution of correlation coefficients and a Dixon range test applied to the transformed values. In the end, however, there is no practical alternative to the average correlation coefficient in the estimate of reference change limits.

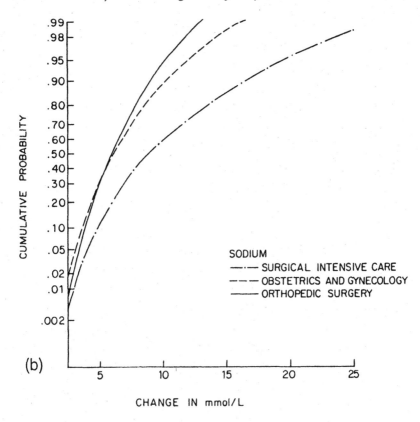

(b)

CHANGE IN mmol/L

urea nitrogen and sodium in each of the three services. Clearly, separate reference change limits are required for each of these services, especially in the surgical intensive care unit.

To compare delta check criteria with reference change limits, Boyd and Harris computed delta values for all seven analytes using nonoverlapping pairs of consecutive determinations. Table 7.2 compares the 2SD limit of the distribution of deltas with $|D_p|$ at four values of p: 0.50, 0.75, 0.90, and 0.95.

In all wards, the delta check limits for both analytes approximated the $|D_{0.50}|$ value except for urea nitrogen in the surgical intensive care unit where the delta check limit was roughly the same as $|D_{0.60}|$. This means that changes exceeding the delta

Table 7.2 Comparison of Reference Change Limits Derived Using the Delta Check Method and the Within-Variances Method

Test and nursing unit	2SD of delta	$|D_p|$ 0.50	0.75	0.90	0.95
Urea nitrogen (mg/L)					
Surgical intensive care	193	133	259	488	710
Orthopedic surgery	54	53	75	102	124
Obstetrics/gynecology	45	46	59	74	85
Sodium (mmol/L)					
Surgical intensive care	8.0	8.9	12.3	16.5	19.6
Orthopedic surgery	5.6	5.9	7.4	9.1	10.2
Obstetrics/gynecology	6.2	6.1	8.1	10.4	12.1

Source: Boyd and Harris (1986), p. 117.

check limit, even if the limit were computed separately for each nursing unit, would be statistically significant at the 5 percent probability level in only about 50 percent of the patients in that nursing unit. The resulting proportion of clinically false positives would undoubtedly be much too high for practical application of these limits in clinical care. Moreover, although the selection of the p value for the reference change limit may vary by ward, depending on experience and the desired clinical sensitivity versus specificity, this method of calculation allows the analyst to estimate the proportion of the target population in whom an observed change exceeding the selected reference change limit would be statistically significant.

7.2.4 Which Variance to Use?

During the last decade, many papers have appeared in the clinical chemistry literature on the estimation of within-subject variance and reference change limits (or critical differences) for analytes in healthy subjects or in groups of patients with different diseases (e.g., Costongs et al., 1985; Hölzel, 1987a,b,c, 1988;

Howey et al., 1987; Gowans and Fraser, 1988; Cummings and Fraser, 1989; Shahangian et al., 1989; Sölétormos et al., 1993; Kairisto et al., 1993; Phillipou and Phillips, 1993). All these authors have tested their data for heterogeneity of within-subject variances (using Bartlett's test), and in many analytes the hypothesis of homogeneity has been rejected. Invariably, however, reference change values have been computed from the average or median value of s_i^2 or from twice the standard deviation of differences between consecutive pairs of observations (delta checking). The alternative procedure described above is usually considered too complicated.[5] This is unfortunate, in our view, because, as noted earlier, the result of applying these published change limits in practice is likely to be a high proportion of reported discrepancies that are not only medically unimportant but not even statistically significant in 40–50 percent of patients. In saying this, we are only repeating Ladenson's remark of 20 years ago (Section 7.2.1) about the "unmanageable" number of discrepancies he encountered when using published estimates of (average) within-subject variances.

Another feature of all these studies except that of Shahangian et al. is that specimens were deep frozen and analyzed in a single run after all had been collected. Thus, between-run analytical variance was eliminated as a component of within-

---

[5] Curiously, Shahangian et al. (1989) used Equation (6.3) to estimate the standard deviation of true within-person variances (σ_i^2) but then calculated reference change limits from selected percentiles of the distribution of observed variances (s_i^2), thereby overestimating these limits (except for that based on the 50th percentile, which is the same for both σ_i^2 and s_i^2). They confirmed the findings of Harris and Yasaka (1983) that in healthy subjects for whom determinations are made at intervals of many months, reference change limits derived from differences between consecutive values correspond to the median within-person variance. As noted earlier, Boyd and Harris (1986) showed that this was also true for delta checks in hospital patients for whom determinations were made every day.

subject variance. As noted earlier, one result of this technique is to underestimate the within-subject variances encountered in real patients whose specimens will be analyzed almost immediately after collection. Between-run analytical variance, if constant during the course of a study, will not affect the estimated variance of σ_i^2; however, eliminating it shifts the proper distribution of $|D_p|$ values to the left, thereby underestimating reference change limits. Resolution of this problem was discussed by Harris and Brown (1979) when the method of reference change limits was introduced.

Costongs et al. (1985) presented critical differences based on both the median and the 90th percentile of observed variances, noting that the former offers greater sensitivity (a smaller critical difference) and the latter, greater specificity. This is true, of course. However, if the observed variances are indeed estimates of a constant within-subject variance in the sampled population, there is no basis in theory for using any statistic other than the mean of the observed variances. On the other hand, if they appear heterogeneous, then, in our view, percentiles of the distribution of true within-subject variances should be sought, as described earlier.

If the heterogeneity of variances is related to the mean values of serial results, as indicated by a plot of s_i^2 versus $\bar{x}_i$, a power or log transformation of the original data may stabilize the variance. If successful, this would greatly simplify calculation of reference change limits, needing only back-transformation of the result to the original scale.

7.3 SUBJECT-SPECIFIC PREDICTIVE VALUES

7.3.1 Introduction

Let us assume that a patient being monitored biochemically appears initially to be in "steady state." In terms of a biochemical analyte, steady state exists when the patient's levels of the analyte are fluctuating over time in random fashion about some homeostatic setpoint specific to the individual. The causes of such fluctuations may be difficult or impossible to identify, but steady state implies that the patient's "system" overcomes their effects and returns the analyte to its setpoint. Neither clinician nor patient would be likely to act until a clinically important change in state occurs and is confirmed. Two general kinds of change are a shift in the setpoint leading to a new steady state, or a continuing trend with no setpoint. Both patient and physician will, of course, be alert to such changes and will want to continue monitoring until the nature and extent of the change become more evident. They will not wait long, however, before intervening to help return the analyte (and the system it represents) to the earlier state. Can statistical methodology provide useful guidelines to aid in confirming the existence of a change?

This is the topic of this section, and it poses something of a dilemma. Should statistical analysis in this situation be restricted to relatively simple methods involving only the sequence of observations in the patient of immediate interest? Alternatively, should more general theory be used to analyze comparable data from a large number of past patients taken as a group, with the information gained from this analysis applied to current patients, treating each separately? Until recently, only the first of these two approaches was available for practical application to patient monitoring, although the general theory mentioned in the alternative has been developing in the statistical literature during the past two decades.

Two common statistical difficulties in patient monitoring are short series in steady state and irregular time intervals between successive measurements. On the other hand, health maintenance programs, aimed at disease prevention or early detection through monitoring healthy subjects and promoting good lifestyles, usually avoid these problems. Since the time intervals are generally much longer in such programs, minor variations can be ignored, while the steady state lasts much longer so that series of moderate length are not uncommon.

The Perfect Liberty health maintenance program in Japan (e.g., Yasaka et al., 1978; Tamura et al., 1987) is a good example, as is the Health Watch program in San Francisco (Williams, 1993), an early and continuing health maintenance program in the United States. Such series of measurements can be managed effectively by relatively simple statistical methods applied to the individual without preliminary examination of multiple series from earlier subjects. We review first some of these methods that appear useful in practice.

7.3.2 Equally Spaced Short Series

The goal of these methods is to use the subject's past series to calculate a predictive range for the current observation. If this observation falls within the range, then it is used to update the range for the next observation. The sequence of measurements may be denoted by $x(1)$, $x(2)$, . . . , $x(t - 1)$, $x(t)$, $x(t + 1)$, ... A simple time series model that has been used to represent steady state in health monitoring programs (e.g., Harris et al., 1980; Albert and Harris, 1987) is the discrete-time first-order autoregressive (AR) model with measurement error:

$$m_{t,i} = \mu_i + \rho_i(m_{t-1,i} - \mu_i) + e_{t,i},$$
$$x_{t,i} = m_{t,i} + a_{t,i}, \tag{7.4}$$

where $m_{t,i}$ and $m_{t-1,i}$ are the unknown circulating (i.e., true) levels of the analyte in the ith subject at the present and just preceding times of measurement; $x_{t,i}$ is the observed value of $m_{t,i}$ with measurement error $a_{t,i}$ including both within-run and between-run analytical inaccuracy; μ_i is the homeostatic set-point around which $m_{t,i}$ is fluctuating; ρ_i, the regression coefficient of $(m_{t,i} - \mu_i)$ on $(m_{t-1,i} - \mu_i)$ and the correlation ($-1 \le \rho_i \le 1$) between successive circulating levels; and $e_{t,i}$, the net effect of biological variability on the current level. Measurement errors are assumed Normally distributed with zero mean and variance σ_a^2, constant for all subjects. Random biological variations during steady state are also assumed Normally distributed with mean zero and variance $\sigma_{e,i}^2$, while $a_{t,i}$ and $e_{t,i}$ are assumed mutually independent and independent of $m_{t,i}$ or any earlier circulating levels or deviations.

An essential characteristic of the discrete-time first-order AR model is that the entire past history of the analyte is incorporated in its state $(m_{t-1,i})$ at the just previous sampling time. However, $m_{t-1,i}$ depends on $m_{t-2,i}$, which depends on $m_{t-3,i}$, etc. If we suppose that the subject's biological state has existed for a very long time, then by repeatedly substituting for m_{t-1} (omitting the subscript i), m_{t-2}, m_{t-3}, etc., in the equation for m_t, the deviation of m_t from its homeostatic setpoint can be expressed entirely in terms of random effects, that is,

$$m_t - \mu = \sum_{j=0}^{\infty} \rho^j e_{t-j} \tag{7.5}$$

This equation implies that the deviation from homeostasis of the circulating level of the analyte at time t is the result of a linear superposition of random biological disturbances, the effect of each declining over time at an exponential decay rate of ρ units per interval. In other words, according to this model, the fluctuation process is entirely stochastic, the cumulative effect of random, independent disturbances.

Further, Equation (7.5) implies that the deviations $(x_t - \mu)$ have a long-term mean of zero and variance

$$\text{Var } x_t = \sigma_x^2 = [\sigma_e^2/(1 - \rho^2)] + \sigma_a^2. \tag{7.6}$$

The variance of the difference between two measurements k time intervals apart is

$$\text{Var } d_k = [2\sigma_e^2(1 - \rho^k)/(1 - \rho^2)] + 2\sigma_a^2. \tag{7.7}$$

From Equations (7.6) and (7.7),

$$\rho = (1/2\alpha)(2 - V_t), \tag{7.8}$$

where $\alpha = 1 - (\sigma_a^2/\sigma_x^2)$, and $V_t = \mathrm{Var}\, d_1/\sigma_x^2$, that is, the ratio of the variance of first differences of the observations to the variance of the observations themselves. Although Equation (7.8) provides only an asymptotic expectation for ρ, it does allow a way of estimating ρ from an observed series.

Since we are concerned at this point with obtaining and updating predictive ranges from the subject's own past data, the general form of the autoregressive model is not immediately practical. At the beginning of monitoring we obviously have insufficient data for estimating ρ. However, after, say, five equispaced observations have been secured while the subject remains in steady state, Equation (7.8) may be used to obtain a crude estimate of ρ from the data (assuming σ_a^2 is known), to be updated as further observations appear. As outlined below, such an estimate can prove useful for continued monitoring.

The simplest form of Equations (7.4), called the *white noise* model, sets $\rho = 0$. That is, the time interval between measurements is supposed to be long enough that the deviation of the previous state from homeostasis has no effect on the current state. This is the model implied in Chapter 6 and behind the calculation of reference change limits where within-subject variance included biological variance plus analytical variance, both within-run and run-to-run. The same result is obtained from Equation (7.7) by setting $\rho = 0$ and $k = 1$. The white noise model allows predictive ranges for a given individual to be developed for unequal as well as equal intervals between observations.

Under this model, the unweighted mean of all past observations, say $\bar{x}_{t-1}$, is the best point estimate of the current observation. The predicted range for this observation is $\bar{x}_{t-1} \pm$ (Student's "t"$_{p,t-2})s_{t-1}[t/(t-1)]^{1/2}$, where s_{t-1} is the standard deviation of past observations of the analyte, while Student's "t" is at significance level p with $t - 2$ degrees of freedom. This formula takes into account both the standard error of the mean and the standard deviation of the present observation, but requires a minimum of four successive observations before it can begin to provide useful forecast ranges. Even then, p should probably be set at 0.1 to reduce the value of "t."

Returning to the general form of the model (Equations 7.4), the optimal predictor of x_t, assuming ρ and μ were known, is $\mu + \rho(x_{t-1} - \mu)$, with mean square error (mse) of prediction $\sigma_x^2(1 - \rho^2)$. However, μ and ρ are unknown, and, in any case, as Cox (1961) has pointed out, if the setpoint has moved from μ to another level, this predictor would be biased and its mse underestimated. Cox investigated the application of a nonparametric, relatively simple, and now widely used method of smoothing and forecasting time series: the exponentially weighted moving average, or ewma, introduced by Holt et al. (1957) and discussed comprehensively by Brown (1962).

The ewma estimate of m_t, the state of the system at time t, puts greatest weight on x_t and exponentially declining weights on earlier observations. This reduces to the recursive form,

$$\hat{m}_t = (1 - \lambda)x_t + \lambda\hat{m}_{t-1}, \tag{7.9}$$

with $\hat{m}_1 = x_1$.

To predict x_t, $\hat{m}_{t-1}$ would be used. However, Cox found that when $\rho \leq \frac{1}{3}$, the *unweighted* mean of past observations is the best predictor of x_t (i.e., the estimate with minimum mse of prediction). Therefore, given the rather long times between observations in typical health monitoring programs, it seems reasonable in this context to begin using the white noise prediction range after four observations have been secured and then test this assumption after the fifth observation by estimating ρ through Equation (7.8).

Cox showed that the ewma worked well as a forecasting procedure for the discrete-time autoregressive model whenever ρ exceeded $\frac{1}{3}$, that is, the mse of one-step-ahead prediction was only slightly higher than if the theoretical predictor could be used. He provided the following formula (Equation 7.10) for the mse of one-step-ahead prediction under this model using the ewma in the presence of measurement error:

$$\text{mse} = \frac{2\sigma_x{}^2(1 - \lambda\rho - \alpha\rho + \alpha\lambda\rho)}{(1 - \lambda\rho)(1 + \lambda)} \qquad (7.10)$$

where α was defined under Equation (7.8).

Remarkably, for a given ρ, it made practically no difference which λ value was used: the mse showed little variation over the entire 0–1 range. However, the mse depended greatly on the value of ρ. When $\alpha = 0.6$ (analytical variance equal to 40 percent of combined analytical plus biological variance), Cox found the unweighted mean of past values to be the optimal predictor whenever ρ was less than 0.455. When analytical variance was 20 percent of total variance ($\alpha = 0.8$), the unweighted mean was best when ρ was less than 0.385.

When ρ approaches its upper bound of unity, the AR model (7.4) converges to a nonstationary model called the random walk. At this point the homeostatic setpoint disappears and the series is characterized by random jumps and apparent but random trends. Although most biochemical analytes in steady state are not likely to exhibit this kind of behavior, some poorly controlled constituents such as metabolic products or triglycerides that are strongly influenced by immediately preceding diet or exercise may conform to a random walk pattern even in steady state (or at least in typical patterns of active, healthy life).

The random walk model has a certain interest for two reasons. First, the ewma is an optimal predictor, not just a good approximation, under the random walk model (Muth, 1960). Second, when the time series appears to be developing a trend of clinical significance, the predictive range for the next observation using the ewma is narrower, and thus more sensitive, than that provided by the white noise model (Harris et al., 1980). Under the random walk model, there is an optimal weight for the ewma, given by

$$w_t = (w_{t-1} + c)/(w_{t-1} + c + 1), \qquad (7.11)$$

where $w_t = 1 - \lambda_t$, $c = \sigma_e{}^2/\sigma_a{}^2$, and $w_1 = 1$ (Stewart, 1970). For $t > 2$ and $c \geq 0.25$, w_t may be set equal to the constant w

$= 1 - \lambda = [-c + \sqrt{(c + 2)^2 - 4}]/2$. The prediction range for the observation x_t becomes $\hat{m}_{t-1} \pm$ (Student's $t_{p,t-2}$) $\sigma_a(\hat{w} + \hat{c} + 1)^{1/2}$. Although x_t is nonstationary under the random walk model, differences between consecutive observations are stationary with mean zero and Var $(d_1) = \hat{\sigma}_e^2 + 2\sigma_a^2$. Therefore, c may be estimated and updated from successive calculations of [Var $(d_1)/\sigma_a^2$] $- 2$, with negative estimates set equal to zero.

Given these various results, a reasonable method for statistical monitoring of equi-spaced observations in a single individual might proceed according to the following steps:

1. Compute means, variances, and the variances of first differences from the beginning of measurement. With only two or three observations, reference change limits may be applied, if available, to judge the difference between successive observations. If the fourth observation appears to be continuing a trend evident in the first three observations, this may be tested for statistical significance using the statistic V_t defined in Equation (7.8). In the presence of a trend, V_t will be small. For $n = 4$, the lower 0.05 and 0.01 percentiles of V_t are 0.780 and 0.626, respectively.[6] If the subject still appears to be in steady state after four observations, use the unweighted mean and standard deviation of these results to calculate a predictive range for the fifth observation.

2. After five observations, estimate the correlation coefficient ρ using Equation (7.8). If $\hat{\rho}$ is less than 0.4, continue to estimate predictive ranges for succeeding observations using the unweighted mean of past values but reestimate ρ after each new observation. If $0.4 \le \hat{\rho} \le 0.9$, use the ewma to compute predictive ranges for the next observation with weight equal, for convenience, to 0.5 (i.e., giving equal weight to the just previous observation and the ewma used to predict that obser-

---

[6] Percentage points of V_t are tabulated in many textbooks. These values were taken from *Documenta Geigy Scientific Tables* (1970), p. 58. The tabled percentage points and underlying theory go back to von Neumann (1941) and Hart (1942).

vation). Estimate the mse for this prediction from Equation (7.10) and calculate the predictive range for x_t as $\hat{m}_{t-1} \pm$ (Student's $t_{p,t-2}$) (mse)$^{1/2}$. In the unlikely case that $\hat{\rho}$ exceeds 0.9, the ewma would be used with λ computed from the random walk formula, Equation (7.11).

3. Continue as long as subject's values remain within predictive ranges, updating mean, variances, and $\hat{\rho}$.

The ewma procedure, unlike the white noise model, requires an estimate of analytical variance (σ_a^2) for the analyte being followed, including, as we mentioned, both within-run and between-run components. These quantities should be available from the laboratory's routine quality control assays. More importantly, neither ρ nor c will be estimated accurately from only a handful of observations. In addition, the ewma method assumes equi-spaced observations. Therefore, in health monitoring programs where long intervals are scheduled between measurements and many years of observation in steady state are not uncommon, the white noise model is probably the most practical (and most likely the optimal) basis for following subjects.

The situation is quite different in patient monitoring where examinations are scheduled at relatively short intervals, but the actual intervals between measurements may vary substantially, while the number of measurements in steady state may be few. Under these circumstances, there is no theory to support subject-specific predictive ranges based solely on the past record of the individual patient.

A recent approach to this problem applies a much more general method of time series analysis to multiple series observed in past patients. Parameters estimated from this analysis are then used to monitor new patients through sequential quality control procedures aimed at flagging observations that indicate significant departures from steady state. In the following section, we describe the main features of this method and the statistical model on which it is based.

7.3.3   Unequally Spaced Short Series

The work referred to has been reported by Schlain et al. (1992, 1993) and rests on a record of publications over many years by Richard Jones (see especially 1981, 1985) concerning estimation of parameters in models of autocorrelated, irregularly spaced data. Other related recent papers are Jones and Ackerson (1990) and Jones and Boadi-Boateng (1991). In the last of these papers, these procedures were applied to serial data on serum creatinine as a function of age in groups of patients with and without a form of kidney disease and with and without hypertension. Schlain et al. extended this methodology by using the estimated parameters to develop a system for flagging atypical observations in new patients, relying on a combination of two well-known sequential quality control procedures: the Shewhart and Cusum techniques.

The contributions of Jones and Ackerson, Jones and Boadi-Boateng, and Schlain et al. refer to a general linear model for longitudinal data developed by Harville (1977) and Laird and Ware (1982). Fixed effects, such as the powers of time in a polynomial growth curve or demographic covariates of the patients, and random effects related to within-patient biological variability and measurement error, are included in this general model, so it is referred to as a mixed model. As Ware (1985) explains, the roots of the proposed model go back many years in statistical research. We define first the elements of this model.

Let n_i be the number of serial measurements of an analyte obtained from the ith patient, and $\mathbf{y}_i$, the $n_i \times 1$ column vector of these measurements. Suppose there are p known constants (e.g., the independent variables in linear regression) associated with each of the measurements. For example, as mentioned earlier, these could be functions of the measurement times, adjusted by subtracting the grand mean of all observation times from each patient's times. Let $\mathbf{X}_i$ be the $n_i \times p$ matrix of these constants, called a *design matrix*, the first column consisting of unities to account for the grand mean of the analyte over all patients. This matrix may also include values of covariates associated with the patient (e.g., see Jones and Boadi-Boateng, 1991). Denote by β the $p \times 1$ vector of fixed, unknown coefficients of these constants, assumed identical for all patients in the same covariate group.

Now introduce γ_i, a $q \times 1$ vector of random effects specific to the ith patient and assumed multiNormally distributed across patients with mean zero and covariance matrix B. Let Z_i be the $n_i \times q$ design matrix for these random effects. For example, in their study of serum creatinine as a function of age in each of four groups of patients, Jones and Boadi-Boateng chose the patient's deviations from the group intercept and group slope as two random effects. Then the first column of Z_i consisted of unities and the second column consisted of the times of each observation.

In addition, there is associated with each patient's measurement a biological "disturbance" $\epsilon_{t,i}$ assumed Normally distributed with mean zero and covariance matrix W_i. Then, the general linear model proposed by Laird and Ware and others to include all of these elements is

$$y_i = X_i\beta + Z_i\gamma_i + \epsilon_{t,i}. \tag{7.12}$$

In applications to biochemical measurements, there is always a measurement error to be included, assumed independent of $\epsilon_{t,i}$ and Normally distributed with variance σ_a^2. This variance is conveniently added to the diagonal elements of W_i. An inital estimate is required, as with the other parameters, but σ_a^2 need not be assumed known; it will be estimated from the likelihood equation.

The great advantage of this model, from the standpoint of patient monitoring, lies in its flexibility to accommodate series that vary in length from one patient to another with variation in the elapsed times between measurements in a given patient. Of particular interest is the use of this model to interpret serial measurements of biochemical tumor markers in patients who have received initial, hopefully curative treatment. For example, Schlain et al. (1992) have applied this model to data from a large sample of patients diagnosed as suffering from stage I or II breast cancer, surgically treated and being followed for possible recurrence. The measured analyte was lipid-associated sialic acid (LSA); log(LSA) was used in the statistical analysis to stabilize the variance across patients. The only within-patient random effect in γ_i was the patient's mean value, and no covariates were included. Therefore, the design matrices X_i and Z_i were both n_i column vectors of unities, β is the (weighted) grand mean of observations over all patients, and B is a scalar denoting the variance of patients' means.

In this study and that of Jones and Boadi-Boateng, the disturbance process $\epsilon_{t,i}$ was treated as a continuous-time first-order autoregressive (CAR) process. A continuous-time process was needed because of the varying time intervals between successive measurements. Applying the CAR model to the biological disturbances represents a fundamental change from the discrete-time autoregressive model given by Equations (7.4) and the accompanying definition of terms. Recall that in discussing this model, we defined the biological disturbances as mutually independent events.

Of course, the mixed model may also be applied to equally spaced observations, as in, for example, Pantula and Pollock (1985), who used a discrete-time AR process to model the disturbance terms. The key question is whether the AR model is being applied to observations in a single individual, as was the case earlier (Section 7.3.2), or whether it is part of a mixed model containing both subject-specific and group parameters. If the latter, we would expect that systematic differences between the ith patient and the average for the group would show up in successive disturbances for that patient that were usually positive or usually negative. In either case, they would be correlated.

Under the CAR process or any stationary model for some time-dependent variable $x(t)$, the autocovariance of values $x(t)$ and $x(t + \tau)$ depends only on the difference τ between the two time points, not on the actual times at which the values occurred. Therefore, for stationary models, the autocovariance may be expressed as $C(\tau)$, and the autocorrelation as $C(\tau)/C(0)$. In the CAR model, $C(\tau) = \sigma^2 e^{-\phi\tau}/2\phi$, where σ^2 is a general variance term and ϕ is often called the autoregression coefficient. The autocorrelation between $x(t)$ and $x(t + \tau)$ is then $e^{-\phi\tau}$. [In Equations (7.4), we used the term $\rho(= e^{-\phi})$ to represent the autocorrelation between values separated by one time unit.] Therefore, apart from the multiplier σ^2, the covariance matrix $\mathbf{W}_i$ of disturbances at observation times t_{ij} and t_{ik} in the ith patient has diagonal elements $[(1/2\phi) + \sigma_a^2]$ and off-diagonal elements given by

$$W_{ijk} = \frac{\exp(-\phi \, |t_{ij} - t_{ik}|)}{2\phi}.$$

Further details of the mathematical procedures used by Jones and Boadi-Boateng and by Schlain et al. to estimate the fixed parameters and the covariance matrices of random effects will not be repeated here. We outline some general directions of these analyses, with particular attention to the work of Schlain et al.

Under the assumptions of Normally distributed random disturbances and measurement errors, and the independence across patients of within-patient random effects, iterative solution of maximum likelihood equations, summed over patients, can be used to obtain estimates of the AR coefficient ϕ, the among-patient variance B, and the variance of measurement error σ_a^2. The iterative process to obtain these estimates over all patients can be combined with calculation of successive expected values and residuals for each individual patient through the use of the Kalman filter. This procedure, now familiar to time series analysts, has been lucidly explained by Meinhold and Singpurwalla (1983). Earlier, Harrison and Stevens (1976) helped to introduce the Kalman filter to statisticians with application to the random walk and other moving average models. A recent text by Shumway (1988, Section 3.4) provides further exposition of the *state-space* methodology involved.

Equations (7.4) represent a simple example of a state-space model where the first equation, the state equation, defines how

m_t, the circulating level of the analyte at time t, is determined from the preceding state m_{t-1} plus a random disturbance. The basic characteristic of the state equation is that it defines the transition from one time to the next of quantities not directly observable. The second equation is called the observation equation. The Kalman filter is a recursive procedure whereby m_t, given the observation y_t, is estimated as the mean of a Bayesian posterior distribution obtained by adjusting the estimate given at the preceding observation ($\hat{m}_t \mid y_{t-1}$), the mean of the Bayesian prior, by the difference (or "residual") between the prior estimate and y_t. At the same time, the variance of the residual is obtained. The current (posterior) estimate then becomes the prior for the estimate of the state at the next time of observation. Let I_t denote the residual $y_t - (\hat{m}_t \mid y_{t-1})$, and V_t, its variance. The process is started with initial estimates of the mean and variance of the state at time zero. The effect of these initial estimates dissipates rapidly as the process moves to later observation times.

The Kalman filter is reinitialized for each patient in the group, but quantities required during the iterative process to obtain maximum likelihood estimates of the "population" parameters (ϕ, B, and σ_a^2) are accumulated over all patients. Jones and colleagues (1990, 1991) computed the variance estimates by first "concentrating out" a general variance term σ^2. Schlain et al. use the same technique, so that the variance parameters B, σ_a^2 and V_t become multiplying factors of σ^2.

The Kalman filter itself is not required to obtain maximum likelihood estimates of the parameters of the mixed model. This is carried out through standard nonlinear optimization procedures within the Kalman filter framework. However, when applied to time series from past patients, estimates of these parameters are not the primary goals of the analysis. The ultimate purpose is to develop reference values for use in monitoring new patients or examining new observations from the original patients. For this purpose, the residuals produced by the Kalman filter for each patient in the study group are the key products, particularly the residuals obtained using the final estimates of the population parameters.

These residuals I_t and their variances V_t are computed for the second and each succeeding observation time of a patient. If the mixed model including the CAR model of the disturbances is an accurate representation of the data, then the standardized variables

$$w_t = I_t/\sigma \sqrt{V_t}$$

based on the maximum likelihood estimates of the CAR parameters are (asymptotically) mutually uncorrelated and Normally distributed with mean zero and unit standard deviation. A test of these conditions is an important part of the computer program. These variables form the basis of the monitoring system used by Schlain et al., the combined Shewhart-Cusum control scheme, introduced by Westgard et al. (1977) for process control in clinical laboratories, and further investigated by Lucas (1982), Yashchin (1985), and others.

A Cusum scheme operates by summing standardized deviations of observed values from the desired value of the process, zero in this case. Usually separate sums are maintained for negative and positive deviations, but one-sided plans maintain only one sum if deviations in only that direction are important. When the cusum is at zero, it will only register a change if the standardized observation is greater than k standard units. This is called the reference value of the scheme. When the cusum exceeds, in absolute value, a selected alarm point h, the system is said to be out of control. The parameters h and k determine the average run length (ARL) of the system: the average number of observations while the system is in control before a false alarm occurs. Formal determination of the ARL requires solution of an integral equation, but tables based on numerical approximations or simulation studies are widely available. Further discussion of Cusum theory may be found in van Dobben de Bruyn (1968). The average run length when the process is not in control depends, of course, on the value of the shift in standard units. The Cusum technique is well known to be highly sensitive to small shifts in mean value away from the desired level.

A combined Shewhart-Cusum scheme adds an additional alarm point, called the Shewhart control limit (C), to the cusum plan so that the process will be considered out of control whenever the cusum exceeds C, usually placed between 3 and 4 standard deviation units. Figure 7.4, taken from Lucas (1982),

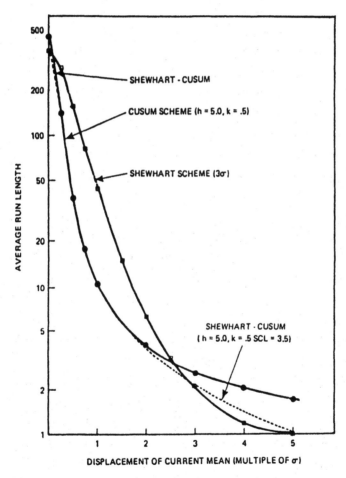

Fig. 7.4   Average run lengths under Shewhart, Cusum, and combined Shewhart-Cusum quality control schemes for increasing shifts of mean value. (From Lucas, 1982, reproduced with permission from the American Society for Quality Control.)

graphs the ARLs for examples of two separate Shewhart and Cusum schemes and a combined scheme when the process is in control and when the mean has been shifted up to 5 standard deviation units.

Schlain et al. (1992) discuss in detail selection of the parameters k, h, and C. To determine the expected performance of a specific Shewhart-Cusum scheme, the authors considered a patient tested every 90 days, a schedule frequently recommended by clinicians. Then, using the final estimates of the CAR parameters and the Kalman filter, they estimate the average standard deviation of residuals in a time series of length 10 at an interval of 90 days between measurements. Next, they suppose two possible alternatives to steady state: one, a 40 percent shift in the standardized residual w after two steady-state test results, followed by successive increases by factors of 1.25 on subsequent tests, and the second, an 80 percent shift beginning at the third and maintained through the fifth test result. With the estimated standard deviation of residuals during steady state, and an alternative to continued steady state specified, formulas are given to calculate the optimal value of k, reasonable values for h and C, and the cumulative probabilities of an alarm signal after the third through sixth test result. These probabilities may then be calculated for alternatives of the same type but with different numerical factors.

The effects of different scheduled intervals between examinations (e.g., 60 rather than 90 days) may be contrasted by repeating this process for each such interval and comparing the corresponding alarm probabilities. Once a set of values for the parameters of the Shewhart-Cusum scheme has been selected, the control scheme may be tried with new patients on their actual time schedule of measurements.

Finally, the authors point out that the reliability of estimated parameters would benefit from periodic repetition of the CAR-Kalman filter analysis, adding steady-state data from new patients and pruning any earlier data found to represent a non–steady-state condition.

This complicated but practical methodology represents, in our view, a major step toward the development of reliable reference values to aid clinicians in the difficult area of patient monitoring, where measurement times are often irregular, series are short, and the need to make timely decisions is urgent. Of course, more experience in applying these methods is necessary as well as user-friendly computer programs that can be widely implemented.

The statistical methods for patient monitoring discussed in this chapter are based largely on random effects, although the mixed model allows for a deterministic function of time as a fixed effect. Many physiological systems and pathological disturbances of these systems have been described mathematically using compartment models involving rates of absorption and elimination. Some of these developments of particular interest to clinical laboratory workers have been summarized by Groth and de Verdier (1982) and Groth (1984), who refers to such models as "biodynamic." In most cases, however, they have not been brought down to the level of individual patient monitoring, where predicted states need to be repeatedly modified by specific patient observations.

One noteworthy exception is therapeutic drug monitoring, where Bayesian forecasting of biochemical analytes in a given patient was pioneered by Sheiner and colleagues (1972, 1977, 1979b). The methodology is similar in many respects to that of Jones and Schlain et al. described above but does not employ the Kalman filter. It is now widely used for monitoring a variety of therapeutic drugs in clinical settings (Sheiner and Ludden, 1992).

A characteristic of the methods discussed above is that the steady state is not expected to be the same in all patients or healthy subjects. Indeed, these dynamic tracking methods should detect early departures from a patient's steady state whatever the average concentration of the analyte may be in that patient. There are, however, two important areas of application of reference values that do not share this basic operational philosophy, where in fact, specific numerical cutpoints are believed by clinicians to have the same diagnostic implications for all patients. One of these, epidemiologically based decision levels for cholesterol, was alluded to in Chapter 1. The other is therapeutic drug monitoring in which the cutpoint is the upper limit of the therapeutic range. These situations raise some particular statistical problems with respect to setting goals for analytical accuracy in the clinical laboratory, the subject of the following two chapters.

APPENDIX 7.1   BASIC PROGRAM FOR REFERENCE CHANGE LIMITS

The first step is to obtain robust estimates of the mean and standard deviation of observed within-subject variances. For this, we include the method of Healy (1979) cited in Section 7.2.2. Sort variances by size and examine the array for possible outliers at either end. Trim the same number of variances, no more than 5 percent, at each end. Find the corresponding unbiasing factor (H), interpolating if necessary, from Table A7.1: Enter the remaining variances from smallest to largest as data in the following program.[7]

Table A7.1

Proportion of variances remaining	H
0.90	2.206
0.92	2.126
0.94	2.046
0.96	1.964
0.98	1.878

Source: Healy (1979, Table 1).

---

[7] The factor 1.28 in statement 370 is the Normal deviate for the 90th percentile of true variances. If another percentile is desired, change 1.28 to the corresponding Normal deviate.

```
10 REM REFERENCE CHANGE LIMITS

20 REM H=HEALY'S UNBIASING FACTOR

30 REM D(I)=ORDERED VARIANCES AFTER TRIMMING

40 REM N=NUMBER OF REMAINING VARIANCES

50 REM M=MEAN OF  LOG VARIANCES

60 REM M1=MEAN OF VARIANCES

70 REM S=EST. VAR. OF LOG VARIANCES

80 REM S1=EST. VAR. OF VARIANCES

90 REM T=EST. VAR. OF TRUE VARIANCES

100 REM V=EST. VAR. OF TRUE LOG VARIANCES

110 REM K=AVERAGE # OBSERVATIONS PER SUBJECT

120 DIM D(50),L(50)

130 H=(to be entered by user)

140 N=(to be entered by user)

150 K=(to be entered by user)

160 OPEN "LPT1:" FOR OUTPUT AS #1

170 M=0

180 W=0

190 FOR I=1 TO N

200 READ D(I)

210 D(I)=LOG (D(I))

220 M=M+D(I)

230 W=W+(D(I))*(2*I-N-1)

240 NEXT I

250 M=M/N
```

```
260 S=W*H/(N*(N-.5))

270 S=S*S

280 M1=EXP(M+(S/2))

290 S1=(M1*M1)*(EXP(S)-1)

300 T=(M1*M1)*(2/(K-1))

310 T=S1-T

320 T=T*((K-1)/(K+1))

330 IF T<0 THEN T=0

340 C=SQR(T)/M1

350 V=T/(M1*M1)

360 V=LOG(V+1)

370 P=M+1.28*SQR(V)

380 R=EXP(P)

390 R=2.77*SQR(R)

400 PRINT #1, "REF. CHANGE LIMIT=",R

410 PRINT #1, "EST. VAR OF TRUE VARIANCES=",T

420 PRINT #1, "EST. CV OF TRUE VARIANCES=",C

430 DATA

440 REM CONTINUE TO END OF DATA

500 END
```

8

ANALYTICAL GOALS FOR REFERENCE VALUES

8.1 INTRODUCTION

Throughout this century, but especially during the post–World War II era, the clinical chemistry profession has mounted a continuing, successful effort to improve the accuracy with which biochemical analytes are measured in the laboratory. During the same period, manufacturers of biochemical analyzers have made great progress in developing more accurate procedures and instruments. Although costs per test have declined, the increasing volume of laboratory analyses has driven higher the total expenditures for biochemical tests.

Some have argued (e.g., Barnett, 1989; Campbell, 1989) that the present state of the art, at least for most quantitative biochemical analyses, has already achieved the accuracy[1] needed for clinical purposes and that any further refinements would not help the physician improve the quality of medical care provided. There is, in short, a "medically acceptable error" for any biochemical analysis, a level of accuracy that has been reached for most analytes, especially those commonly requested by clinicians.

The issue of whether the accuracy of existing analytical methods in clinical laboratories is adequate to meet medical needs is central to a discussion of analytical goals. It has been increasingly studied and discussed in the clinical chemistry and pathology literature. There seem to be essentially two problems

---

[1] We use the words *accuracy* and *inaccuracy* in this chapter to connote the agreement or lack thereof between a laboratory measurement of a biochemical analyte and the "true" value of that analyte. This definition is consistent with that used, for example, by Westgard et al. (1974), who also cite the same usage in much earlier writings on measurement and testing. Other authors, ourselves included, have often used inaccuracy in a more restricted sense to refer only to the "systematic bias" of a measurement system, in contrast to its "imprecision." (The words *true* value, *systematic bias*, and *imprecision* are defined in statistical terms later in the text). As Westgard et al. pointed out, the definition of accuracy employed here conforms to the operational understanding of the term by clinicians.

involved. The first is to determine the numerical guidelines that physicians follow when interpreting the results of laboratory analyses in various clinical situations. The second is to translate these guidelines into standards of analytical accuracy that clinical laboratories should satisfy.

The first problem clearly requires the cooperation of clinicians and probably leadership by physicians, especially clinical pathologists, although some pioneering work in this area has been carried out by a nonphysician (Elion-Gerritzen, 1980). The second problem will probably be resolved most satisfactorily by a combination of statistical modeling and experience in the procedures used in clinical laboratories to maintain analytical accuracy. The last few years have seen some important contributions to a solution of this problem. These will be discussed in Section 8.3 together with studies of clinicians' practices in the interpretation of biochemical test results.

This chapter will focus on several general contexts in which biochemical reference values are used as guidelines in reaching clinical decisions. In each context, there are biological as well as analytical sources of variation that influence the difference between an observed value and the reference value. In healthy subjects, some sources of within-subject biological variation, such as the physiological condition of the person at the time the blood or other fluid specimen is drawn (so-called pre-analytical variation) can be controlled by following well-defined rules of patient behavior prior to sampling (e.g., IFCC, Part 3, 1988). Other rules concern the procedures for securing and handling the specimen before analysis.

These pre-analytical rules have been formulated because studies have shown (e.g., Statland et al., 1973; Statland and Winkel, 1981) that they are needed to protect the accuracy of the measured value. If values from different subjects are aggregated into a collective from which a population-based reference range is calculated, application of these rules helps to reduce sampling "noise" that unnecessarily widens the range. The rules serve the same purpose when the difference between two observations is used to judge whether a medically important change has occurred in the patient's condition.

Biological variation among reference subjects can be reduced somewhat (but usually not much) by deliberate selection of subjects according to demographic or other characteristics determined beforehand. In Chapter 6, we examined this possibility and provided some criteria for judging whether or not separate reference ranges should be developed for different population subgroups. In the end, however, the appropriate level of accuracy for the biochemical analysis itself remains a key issue.

In agreement with many clinical chemists and others who have investigated this topic, we look at analytical variation in relation to biological variability. The kinds of biological variation involved will differ from one context of use of reference values to another. Therefore, in our view, the issue concerns the maximum allowable analytical variation relative to biological variation in any context of use of reference values.

Two sources contribute to analytical inaccuracy: imprecision and bias. The former is defined as the difference between the measured value of some quantity (e.g., the concentration of a biochemical constituent in a given matrix) and the mean [or expected value, $E(x)$] of a large number of such measurements. The difference is presumed due to the net effect of many unpredictable, randomly occurring influences. Imprecision is thus assumed to be a statistically random variable with mean zero and variance commonly denoted by σ_a^2, a usage employed in earlier chapters.

In clinical laboratory practice, σ_a^2 is further specified as either "between-runs" (i.e., "run-to-run") or "within-run" variance. Between-run variance includes components of variance due to changes in analytic conditions (some identifiable, some not) that are kept effectively constant within a "run" of measurements. Examples of identifiable factors are changes in batches of reagents or in calibrating materials. The collection of measurements from a group of reference subjects (blood donors, for example, or outpatients at a selected clinic) usually requires considerable time and many analytical runs. Similarly, monitoring a patient in steady state usually implies a fairly long time interval between measurements. Therefore, in setting goals for analytical precision, we should be concerned with placing limits on long-term variance, combining both within- and between-run variance components.

In addition, σ_a^2 is commonly found to depend on the true concentration of the analyte. We mentioned this in Chapter 2 as one of the factors inducing positive skewness in the distribution of cross-sectional reference values. Often the coefficient of variation (CV) is more constant than the variance across a range of concentrations; in any case, CV is a nondimensional parameter that can be compared for many analytes. For this reason (100 CV_a) percent is typically used as the measure of imprecision.

Bias is the difference between the mean value of a large number of replicate measurements and the "true" value of the quantity being measured. We identify the latter as the concentration of the biochemical constituent in a specimen of blood (or other body fluid) at the time the specimen is presented to the measurement system for analysis.[2] Then, a nonzero bias reflects a defect in the analytical specificity of the measuring system, due often to the effects of other substances present in the specimen that interfere with the measurement procedure.

Within the laboratory, the bias of a new measuring system may be estimated from percentage recoveries of known amounts of the analyte in a suitable matrix. In routine use, both bias and imprecision are monitored within and across runs by testing known control samples such as specimens from a frozen serum pool or dilutions of lyophilized (dried) analyte material in an appropriate solvent.

---

[2] In Chapter 7, we used the words "circulating" value to indicate the "true" value of the analyte. The circulating value would be the same as the value presented to the measurement system if the net effect of procedures used to obtain and handle the specimen prior to analysis did not alter the concentration.

Bias may also be estimated by comparing the measurements of specimens at different concentrations split between the test system and a definitive (or "reference") system believed to be free of bias. The usual procedure is to regress test measurements against reference measurements by ordinary least squares. If the fitted straight line appears to go through the origin (e.g., by statistical test of the estimated intercept), the test system is said to have zero *systematic* bias. Otherwise, such bias is a negative or positive amount. If the slope of the line differs significantly from unity, the test system is said to have *proportional* bias; that is, the extent of the difference between the mean of replicate measurements and the true concentration depends on the true value.

Bias estimated through comparison of a test system with a definitive procedure is a fundamental characteristic of the test system. There are other sources of intermittent bias between runs that are attributable not to the biochemical principles of the measurement procedure but to identifiable changes in analytical conditions. As we noted earlier, such temporary biases are included in the definition of between-run imprecision. Finally, since clinical decisions often center on specific concentrations (e.g., upper or lower reference limits or other cutpoints), we assume that the goals for reducing inaccuracy refer to measurements in the neighborhood of these critical decision points. The acceptable bias or imprecision of a measurement system might then be expressed as a percentage of the critical reference value.

To summarize, total analytical error (TAE) or inaccuracy in the clinical laboratory analysis of a body fluid constituent is the difference between the measured value of the analyte (x) and its true value (μ). In statistical terms,

$$TAE = x - \mu = [(x - E(x)] + [E(x) - \mu], \qquad (8.1)$$

where E stands for expected (or mean) value. The variance of TAE, say, σ_T^2, is obtained by squaring both sides of the second equation and taking expected values. Thus,

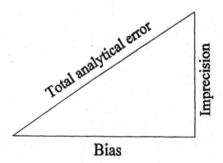

Fig. 8.1 Right triangular relation connecting imprecision, bias, and total analytical error. (Adapted from Deming, 1950, p. 129.)

$$\sigma_T^2 = \sigma_a^2 + B^2, \tag{8.2}$$

where B, the bias term, is $E(x) - \mu$.[3]

Equation (8.2) is a right-triangular relation connecting the standard deviation of TAE, the standard deviation of imprecision σ_a, and the bias B of a system of analytical measurement. This fundamental relation is pictured in Figure 8.1. Equation (8.2) is used in some of the approaches to analytical goals discussed below, but more often attention has been given to models defining TAE without extension to its variance.

8.2 ANALYTICAL GOALS FOR GROUP-BASED REFERENCE RANGES

The recent literature on the issue of analytical goals as they relate to the use of reference values in clinical practice has, to

---

[3] To distinguish within- and between-run imprecision, σ_a^2 might be subdivided into two components, $\sigma_{a(w)}^2$, the variance of measurements of control samples within a run, and $\sigma_{a(b)}^2$, the variance of run means around the expected value $E(x)$. To avoid further multiplicity of subscripted symbols, we have not used this notation but define the analytical variance component referred to in each context.

a large extent, coalesced into reviews and published proceedings of conferences. In particular, excellent reviews by Fraser (1981, 1983) have clarified and summarized various competing concepts and arguments about analytical goals up to the beginning of the last decade. Fraser also included the recommendations of the first general symposium on the subject of analytical goals in clinical chemistry, the 1976 Aspen conference sponsored by the College of American Pathologists (CAP) (1977). A follow-up conference in 1978, sponsored by the World Association of Societies of Pathology (1979), supported the recommendations of the Aspen symposium.

A subsequent conference in 1987, again under the aegis of the CAP (1988), was primarily concerned with evaluating results of the laboratory proficiency testing program of the CAP but also contained a number of presentations relevant to the subject of analytical goals. Finally, in 1992, the American Association of Clinical Chemists sponsored a forum on analytical goals and medical relevance (1993). In addition to these American-sponsored conferences (which drew many participants from other countries), the Nordic Clinical Chemistry Project (NORDKEM), founded in 1977 by the Nordic Council of Ministers "to promote the quality of performance in hospital laboratories in the Nordic countries," has published several monographs (1980, 1984, 1992) that include many contributions to the subject of this chapter.

The earliest recommended general formula for allowable analytical error appears to be that of Tonks (1963), although this author cites specific numerical values used by previous writers. Tonks proposed that TAE (in percent) should not exceed one-quarter of the "normal range" divided by the "mean" (presumably, the midpoint) of the range, multiplied by 100. Campbell and Owen (1967) and Fraser (1981, and later writings) have criticized the use of the reference range as the basis for setting a limit to TAE because the range includes analytical imprecision. Therefore, if it were based on measurements with a high (low) amount of imprecision, the allowable TAE would also be high (low).

In fact, Tonks's selection of the factor $\frac{1}{4}$ to apply to the reference range is rather strange in itself. For symmetric or mildly skewed distributions, the width of the 95 percent reference range is approximately $4\sqrt{(\sigma_a^2 + \sigma_b^2)}$, where σ_b^2 represents combined within- and among-subject biological variance. Thus, allowing σ_a to be as large as one-quarter of the reference range requires that the range be derived from data whose imprecision is already much less than the allowable limit, for otherwise there would be no room left for biological variation!

The basic flaw in Tonks's formula is not its somewhat circular argument in appealing to the reference range, although this criticism is warranted, but rather that it fails to take account of existing biological variance when deciding on the allowable level of analytical variance. Consider, for example, the context of diagnostic screening, that is, deciding on the basis of a single measurement whether or not the patient is harboring a given disease. This is the traditional and most appropriate application of population-based reference ranges. In this context, combined within- and among-subjects biological variance represents a major and unchangeable contribution to the width of a reference range. Analytical variance, on the other hand, is an artifactual contribution that may be reduced or increased by practices and conditions within the laboratory. In deciding on a limit to analytical variance, it seems sensible to choose this limit in relation to the size of the basic component of total variance, namely, biological variance.

With this in mind, Cotlove et al. (1970) recommended that for purposes of diagnostic screening, analytical variation σ_a should not exceed one-half the combined within- and among-subjects biological variation σ_b. The rationale for the factor $\frac{1}{2}$ was that such a level of σ_a would not extend the reference range by more than 12 percent over what its width would be in the absence of analytical variation. That is, if $\sigma_a \leq \frac{1}{2}\sigma_b$, then $\sqrt{(\sigma_a^2 + \sigma_b^2)} \leq 1.12\sigma_b$. Cotlove et al. recognized that patient monitoring would require a more stringent limit on analytical variation because in this context only within-subject biological variation is involved. Therefore, they suggested that for this purpose, σ_b should represent average within-subject variation.

Turning back to Table 6.2, which summarized analytical and biological CV's for many analytes, we find as of that date (1982) that long-term analytical variation was less than half the average within-subject biological variation in only eight of twenty commonly measured analytes: triglyceride, uric acid, bilirubin, urea nitrogen, phosphorus, creatine kinase, iron, and potassium. In several of these, within-subject variation is well known to be large, because of variations in diet and exercise. When within-subject and among-subjects variances are combined into a single term, the number of analytes for which analytical variation failed to satisfy the Cotlove rule drops from twelve to six: creatinine, calcium, albumin, thyroxine, sodium, and chloride.

The Aspen conference accepted the proposal of Cotlove et al. and proceeded to publish numerical limits for σ_a in many analytes commonly measured in the clinical laboratory. These limits were drawn from studies of within- and among-subjects variances in healthy individuals summarized by Statland and Winkel at the Aspen conference and reported previously in the clinical chemistry literature (e.g., Statland et al. 1973, 1974; Winkel et al., 1975).

Fraser has argued that the more stringent goal, $\sigma_a \leq$ half the average within-subject biological variation, should be adopted on the ground that a laboratory analysis should be sufficiently precise to satisfy its most demanding use. Moreover, as Fraser (1988) has pointed out (also see Fraser and Harris, 1989; Fraser and Petersen, 1993), there is now considerable evidence of stability in average within-subject standard deviation regardless of age, geographic location, time span of the study (beyond a week), or whether the individual is healthy or burdened by chronic but stable disease.

Since the limits on σ_a proposed by Cotlove et al. refer only to analytical imprecision, they cannot represent limits on TAE unless one assumes that bias should be reduced to zero. In fact, until the late 1980s, little attention was paid in the clinical chemistry literature to the question of goals for analytical bias, then usually called analytical "inaccuracy." A notable exception is the landmark paper by Westgard et al. (1974). Authors generally believed that bias could and should be reduced to zero. With the advent of definitive methods for measuring analytes commonly ordered by clinicians, the biases of field methods for these analytes (i.e., methods practical for widespread use but usually based on less specific biochemical procedures) could be reliably estimated. Methods with clearly unacceptable biases were rapidly replaced by improved systems. It became recognized, however, that existing biases in methods widely used in clinical laboratories might never (or only very slowly) be entirely eliminated. Recently, therefore, greater attention has been devoted to establishing goals for analytical bias as well as imprecision.

In 1988, Gowans et al. computed the effects of different combinations of imprecision σ_a and systematic (i.e., constant) bias B, relative to combined biological variation σ_b on the probability of false-positive decisions in diagnostic screening. It is instructive to consider each type of error separately, then put them together into a single formula.

In the absence of any form of analytical error, and assuming a Normal distribution of reference values, 2.5 percent of healthy subjects will show test values outside the (true) upper reference limit $\mu + 1.96\sigma_b$. Under these idealized conditions, taking the upper reference limit as the diagnostic decision point, 0.025 is the probability of a false-positive diagnosis in favor of a disease presumed to increase the level of the analyte. Suppose now that analytical imprecision with standard deviation $\sigma_a = 0.5\sigma_b$ is added, the maximum recommended by Cotlove et al., increasing the overall standard deviation by a factor of 1.12. This widens the reference distribution so that the old reference limit is now (1.96/1.12), or 1.75 standard deviations above the mean, and cuts off 4.0 percent of the reference population. The probability of false-positive diagnosis has increased by 60 percent although the absolute change may seem small, 1.5 percent. In fact, looked at in this way, the Cotlove limit does not seem too stringent.

In general, if imprecision with standard deviation $\sigma_a = k\sigma_b$ is added, the new standard deviation of the reference distribution will be $\sigma' = (1 + k^2)^{1/2}\sigma_b$, and the location of the original 97.5 percent reference limit will now be $1.96/(1 + k^2)^{1/2}$ standard deviations above μ.

Suppose that a positive bias of $B = m\sigma_b$ is added. This changes the position of the mean to $\mu' = \mu + B$. The combined effect of the added bias and imprecision is to convert the original reference distribution to a new Normal distribution with mean μ' and standard deviation σ'. With respect to this distribution, the original 97.5 percent reference limit will be located at the point $z_0 = (1.96 - m)/(1 + k^2)^{1/2}$ standard deviations from the mean. The probability of false-positive diagnosis, say P_f is then given by

$$P_f = 1 - \int_{-\infty}^{z_0} \phi\,(z)\,dz, \tag{8.3}$$

where $\phi(z)$ denotes the standard Normal density function. For example, if $k = 0.5$ and $m = 0.3$, the original decision point will be 1.482 standard deviations from the mean, and the rate of false-positive decisions will have increased to 6.9 percent, or almost triple the original rate in the absence of analytical error.

Negative bias $(-m)$ pushes the original reference limit farther out on the right-hand tail of the distribution, thus decreasing the rate of false positives in that direction but increasing the probability of false negatives. Figure 8.2, from the work of Gowans et al. (1988), pictures the rising rates of false-positive diagnoses as the standard deviation of imprecision (σ_a, relative to σ_b) increases for different amounts of systematic bias in screening against a disease that induces high values of the analyte. For example, restricting P_f to 5 percent and imprecision to the extent of $\sigma_a = 0.5\sigma_b$ (where σ_b includes both within- and among-subjects biological variation) limits the bias of the measuring system to approximately 10 percent of σ_b.

Also included in Figure 8.2 is a semicircle representing a suggestion by Harris (1988) that the Cotlove rule ($\sigma_a \leq \frac{1}{2}\sigma_b$) be extended to include bias; that is, following Equation (8.2), setting $\sigma_T = (\sigma_a{}^2 + B^2)^{1/2} \leq \frac{1}{2}\sigma_b$, or $(k^2 + m^2)^{1/2} \leq \frac{1}{2}$.

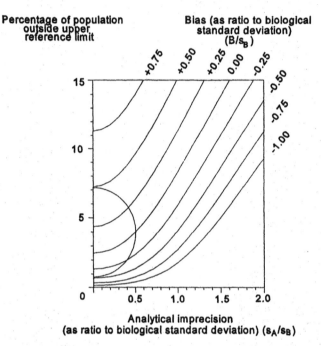

Fig. 8.2 Expected proportions of population outside upper reference limit for increasing amounts of imprecision and bias. (From Gowans et al., 1988, with permission.) Semicircle insert represents rule of Cotlove et al. (1970) (see text).

The effect of systematic bias on the probability of false-positive diagnosis is much greater than a comparable degree of analytical imprecision. For example, as calculated earlier, when $k = 0.5$ in the absence of bias, P_f is increased by 60 percent. However, when $m = 0.5$ while $k = 0$, P_f is increased by 189 percent.

As noted, these calculations assume a Normal reference distribution, either on the original or transformed scale. If a transform of scale is required, then both analytical and biological variances must be estimated on this scale (Petersen et al., 1989). Finally, the presence of proportional bias would make the bias at critical decision points less or greater than systematic bias alone. Similarly, assay imprecision may not be constant along the reference range. Transformation, if necessary, to a Normally distributed measurement scale should reduce or eliminate such features, but, in any case, our interest is in the analytical error at the reference limit or other decision point.

The work of Gowans et al. (1988) was motivated by a desire to investigate analytical goals when reference ranges are to be established by a national laboratory from a large number of selected subjects and then distributed to regional laboratories for local use. This would have many potential advantages in a small country of fairly homogeneous biological stock; in particular, the authors consider Scotland and Denmark, their home-lands, as examples. The authors' methods for dealing with this special problem are not described here, but we note that they lead to stricter bounds on imprecision and bias, considered jointly, than other proposed limits (e.g., Harris, 1988).

The equations and computations presented so far concern the limits on analytical imprecision and bias needed to satisfy a specified probability of false-positive diagnosis in a screening situation where the decision points are the upper (or lower) limits of the 95 percent reference range. A full study of the effects of analytical imprecision and bias on the efficiency of diagnostic screening must include information on the distribution of the analyte in the diseased population, the prevalence of the disease, the costs of false-positive and false-negative decisions, the gains of true-positive decisions, and the costs of improved analytical accuracy. With this information, an optimal decision point can be determined and changes in total costs plotted as a function of analytical imprecision and bias. This is clearly a considerable undertaking. An exceptional example has been provided by Groth et al. (1983) in screening patients for hyperparathyroidism through measurement of serum calcium.

Figure 8.3, taken from Petersen and Hørder (1988), illustrates the general effects of analytical imprecision and bias on the probabilities of false-positive and false-negative decisions

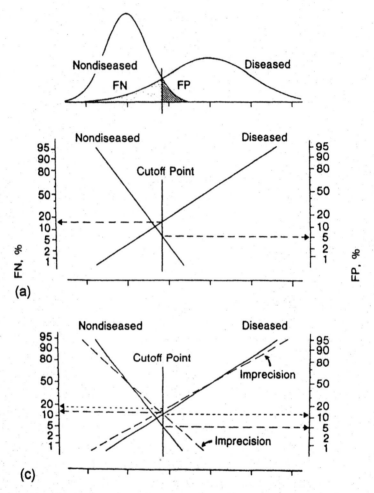

Fig. 8.3 Effects of bias and imprecision on false negative (*FN*) and false positive (*FP*) decisions in diagnostic screening. (a) no analytical error; (b) positive bias, no imprecision; (c) imprecision, no bias; (d) positive bias and imprecision. In (a), (b), and (c), long horizontal dashes indicate absence of analytical error. (From Petersen and Hørder, 1988, Copyright 1988, American Medical Association.)

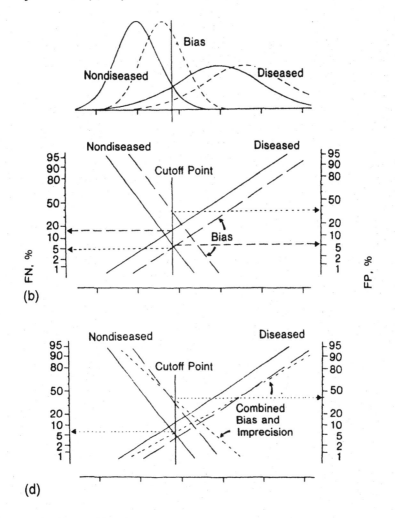

in diagnostic screening. Normal distributions of an analyte in diseased and nondiseased populations are plotted on cumulative probability scales, converting the distributions to straight lines. The diseased population is cumulated in the usual way from low to high values; the nondiseased population is cumulated in reverse, from high to low. The effect of analytical imprecision is to increase the spread of the distributions without changing the discrimination point, thereby increasing the probabilities of both types of diagnostic errors (decreasing both sensitivity and specificity).[4] Positive bias is equivalent to a displacement of the discrimination point to the left, increasing sensitivity but decreasing specificity; negative bias produces the reverse effect. The net effect of both sources of analytical error is pictured in the bottom right graph.

In the diagnostic screening context, biological variation is defined to include both within-subject and among-subjects variability. In the next two sections, we discuss clinical uses of reference values that involve only within-subject biological variance. In these contexts, information on perceived medical needs plays a major role in determining appropriate analytical goals. Such information might be obtained, for example, by surveying the opinions of clinicians or from the recommendations of a body of physicians guided by epidemiological data.

8.3 ANALYTICAL GOALS IN DETECTING PATIENT CHANGES

The need to take medical relevance into account when setting analytical goals becomes most apparent when laboratory tests are used in patient management. The attending physician is clearly responsible for deciding whether an observed change between two successive results in a patient warrants further action (e.g., ordering another test, changing the dosage of a drug, or starting a new course of therapy).

The main focus in this section will be on statistical models for determining analytical goals when reference values are used in the context of patient monitoring. The most recent of these models attempt to take account of the numerical criteria used by clinicians to evaluate observed changes in test results. The relatively few studies of this subject (Skendzel, 1978; Barrett et

---

[4] *Clinical sensitivity* is defined as the probability that individuals with the disease will exhibit a test value outside the reference value. *Clinical specificity* is the probability that individuals free of the disease will present a value inside the reference value.

al., 1979; Elion-Gerritzen, 1980; Skendzel et al., 1985; and Thue et al., 1991) have used questionnaires to survey the opinions of clinicians concerning the changes in test values they would regard as worthy of medical action in patients with specific medical problems.

In the most extensive of these studies, that of Skendzel et al. (1985), a series of vignettes were posed, each concerning a hypothetical patient, usually with a specific clinical problem but also including the individual without complaints who comes in for routine physical checkup. The physician was presented with an initial value (sometimes the upper or lower limit of the reference range) for a given analyte and asked to select the closest value that would signify a change warranting medical action. The sampling was nationwide, and returns were received from 745 clinicians, including specialists as well as family practitioners.

All of these studies have shown that physicians are highly variable in their opinions about the smallest change they would tolerate in a given analyte before intervening.[5] This is not surprising because physicians differ in their knowledge of and the consideration they give to the many causes of variability in biochemical test results, including nonuniform pre-analytical conditions and within-subject biological variation. In addition, the critical changes reported for a given analyte depend on the clinical situation.

To utilize the information obtained from surveys of clinicians' opinions, arbitrary decisions have to be made, as is inevitable regardless of which path is taken to derive analytical goals. Skendzel et al. chose to report the median value of the smallest change in test results labeled medically significant by the responding clinicians. These medians were converted to concentration ratios, dividing in most cases by the upper limit of the reference range. Finally, a "medically useful coefficient of variation," recommended as an appropriate goal for analytical preci-

---

[5] Skendzel (1978) recorded this variability, but it was not included in the report by Skendzel et al. (1985).

sion, was computed by dividing the ratio by the Normal deviate 1.645 or $1.645\sqrt{2}$, depending on whether the initial value was considered a fixed standard (e.g., the upper limit of a reference range) or a test value subject to analytical error.

The rationale for this calculation lies in the following argument. If, in fact, there is no change between the true analyte values on two successive occasions, and if the only reason an observed change is not zero is because of analytical imprecision, then such observed changes should be Normally distributed with mean zero and standard deviation σ_a. A "medically useful" value for σ_a would be such that only 5 percent of observed changes (when the true change is zero) exceed the median smallest value warranting medical action, as judged by clinicians. Hence, dividing this median value (or its concentration ratio) by $1.645\sqrt{2}$ yields the recommended goal for σ_a (or its corresponding CV).

This reasoning was critically examined in the two modeling efforts described next. The median "just medically significant" values reported by Skendzel et al. were retained, but were used in different ways.

8.3.1 Modeling by Linnet

Linnet (1989) pointed out that analytical imprecision is not the only cause of fluctuations in serial test results around a true steady state. Within-patient biological variation and pre-analytical variation also contribute and must be allowed for, placing more stringent requirements on purely analytical error if the medically useful criterion is to be met.[6] Therefore, Linnet replaced the "medically useful" CV of Skendzel et al. by a CV including all these sources of variation that may be written

---

[6] The study of clinical opinions by Thue (1991) did take account of biological variation in computing medically important CV's. However, this study was restricted to hemoglobin and included a smaller sample of physicians. It is a good model for wider investigations of clinicians' interpretation of observed changes.

$$C_t = (C_p{}^2 + C_a{}^2 + C_b{}^2)^{1/2},$$

where the subscript p refers to pre-analytical variation. Linnet set C_p equal to half C_a (citing the relevant sources for this), so that the formula for total CV becomes

Table 8.1 CV's (%) of Analytical Imprecision (C_a), Within-subject Biological Variation (C_b), and Total (C_t) Compared to Median "Just Medically Significant" Change (Δ_{med})

Analyte	C_a	C_b	$C_t{}^a$	$\Delta_{med}{}^b$	$\Delta_{med}/$ $(C_t\sqrt{2})$
Aspartate transaminase	8.7	16.0	18.2	33.3	1.29
Bilirubin	9.2	25.0	26.6	12.6	0.33
Calcium	2.2	1.4	2.6	11.2	3.05
Cholesterol	3.9	5.4	6.7	28.6	3.02
Creatinine	6.8	4.6	8.2	16.6	1.43
Glucose	3.4	6.2	7.1	26.1	2.60
Iron	4.6	27.0	27.4	40.0	1.03
Phosphorus	3.0	7.8	8.4	33.3	2.80
Potassium	1.9	5.1	5.4	11.2	1.47
Sodium	1.1	0.74	1.3	4.0	2.18
Thyroxine	7.7	8.8	11.7	40.0	2.42
Total protein	2.3	2.7	3.5	19.3	3.90
Triglyceride	5.3	27.0	27.5	37.4	0.96
Urea nitrogen	4.5	13.0	13.8	20.1	1.03

[a] Computed according to Equation (8.4).
[b] These values have been derived from the data in Tables 1 and 2 of Skendzel et al. In the great majority of cases, these authors computed their medically useful CV's by dividing Δ_{med} by $1.645\sqrt{2}$, assuming both test values subject to analytical error. In these instances, therefore, we multiplied the CV of Skendzel et al. by this factor to retrieve Δ_{med}. In the remaining examples, the authors divided by 1.645, taking the initial value to be a fixed reference point not subject to error. In these cases, we multiplied by this factor to obtain Δ_{med}. Where Skendzel et al. listed several values for a given analyte, corresponding to different clinical situations, we have chosen the smallest value of Δ_{med} on the ground that analytical error should be low enough to satisfy the most demanding clinical requirement. For these reasons, the values of Δ_{med} listed in this table differ somewhat from those in Linnet's paper (Table 1).

$$C_t = (1.25 \, C_a{}^2 + C_b{}^2)^{1/2}. \qquad\qquad (8.4)$$

Linnet tabulated numerical values for these CV's in the manner of Table 8.1, using figures from the Aspen conference report and CAP surveys, then compared C_t to the median "just significant" changes (Δ_{med}) reported by Skendzel et al. For consistency, Table 8.1 includes CV's for analytical and within-subject biological variation taken from Table 6.2; the numbers are similar to those used by Linnet.

For seven of the fourteen analytes listed (AST, bilirubin, creatinine, iron, potassium, triglyceride, and urea nitrogen), the last column of Table 8.1 falls below 1.65. In all of these analytes except creatinine, the average within-person biological CV (C_b) is so large that even if C_a were reduced to zero, $\Delta_{med}/C_b\sqrt{2}$ would still fall below 1.65. One may conclude that in many clinical situations, clinicians underestimate the biological variation associated with the analyte, perceiving as critical changes that in reality are too small to warrant immediate medical action. Linnet remarks on this particularly with respect to iron and triglyceride.

Linnet argued, moreover, that even for those analytes whose analytical imprecision appears to satisfy the median medically useful CV, the clinical laboratory must remain vigilant to detect the occurrence of bias or out-of-control imprecision that would undermine this usually satisfactory level of accuracy. He defined a maximally allowable systematic bias (ΔSE_c) that would artifactually shift the patient's baseline upwards but fall just short of producing a false-positive change, using Δ_{med} as the criterion. That is, the distance between a true change of zero and Δ_{med} has been shortened by ΔSE_c, but remains at the borderline $1.645\sqrt{2}C_t$, maintaining a 5 percent probability of false-positive decision. In symbols,

$$\Delta_{med} - \Delta SE_c = 1.645\sqrt{2}C_t,$$

or

$$\Delta SE_c = \Delta_{med} - 1.645\sqrt{2}C_t. \qquad\qquad (8.5)$$

Similarly, Linnet considered the possibility of an out-of-control deterioration in analytical precision that would increase the CV of imprecision from C_a to C_a' and C_t to C_t', so that whereas $\Delta_{med}/(\sqrt{2}C_t)$ exceeded 1.645, now $\Delta_{med}/(\sqrt{2}C_t')$ just equals 1.645. Then, assuming pre-analytical variation remains the same,

$$C_t' = \Delta_{med}/1.645\sqrt{2},$$

whence

$$C_a' = (C_t'^2 - C_b^2 - 0.25\,C_a^2)^{1/2}. \tag{8.6}$$

Linnet's thesis is that the laboratory's quality control procedures must be sufficiently powerful (preferably with a probability of 90 percent or more) to detect the maximal levels of bias and increase in imprecision. These maximal levels computed from Table 8.1 for those analytes satisfying Skendzel's criterion (calcium, cholesterol, glucose, phosphorus, sodium, thyroxine, and total protein) are listed in Table 8.2, where ΔSE_c and C_a' have been standardized to nondimensional units by dividing by C_a (following Linnet).

Table 8.2 Standardized Maximal Allowable Levels of Bias and Increase in Imprecision to Meet Most Stringent Medically Useful CV (Δ_{med}) Reported by Skendzel et al. (1985)

Analyte	$\Delta SE_c/C_a$	C_a'/C_a
Calcium	2.3	2.0
Cholesterol	3.3	2.8
Glucose	2.8	2.7
Phosphorus	4.6	4.0
Sodium	0.89	1.3
Thyroxine	1.7	1.9
Total protein	4.9	3.4

Linnet reviewed the power of various quality control rules (Westgard and Groth, 1979; Westgard and Barry, 1986). He found that to achieve a power of detection close to or above 0.9, even when standardized maximal bias or imprecision equals or exceeds 3, a multi-rule must be followed with at least two control samples per run. For standardized maximal errors up to about 2, the power is less than 0.5 under all except the multi-rule with at least four control samples per run. Thus, for sodium and thyroxine (Table 8.2), no reasonable quality control rule offers good power to detect an analytical error that would cause a test result to fail to meet Skendzel's criterion of medical usefulness.

In short, for at least nine of the fourteen common analytes listed in Table 8.1, Linnet's statistical models show that either (1) present-day analytical imprecision and bias should be reduced to assure (with 90 percent probability) that changes in test results perceived as medically significant by 50 percent of clinicians in typical patient situations would in fact not be false positives, or (2) these just significant changes are really too narrow (at least, the strictest ones), perhaps because clinicians fail to take sufficient account of within-patient biological variability.

By extending Linnet's findings a little, we reach another interesting conclusion. Suppose the standardized maximal errors $\Delta SE_c/C_a$ and C'_a/C_a are both set equal to 3, the least value that affords good power of error detection at a probability of false positive around 0.05 under a reasonable quality control rule (Linnet, 1989, Table 3). Then, eliminating Δ_{med}/C_a between Equations (8.5) and (8.6) and solving for the ratio C_a/C_b, we obtain a result approximately equal to 0.5, the goal for analytical imprecision recommended by Cotlove et al.[7] Thus, this goal, developed originally without reference to medically significant changes in test results or to the power of detecting out-of-con-

---

[7] If both $\Delta SE_c/C_a$ and C'_a/C_a are set equal to a constant K, a good approximation for C_a/C_b when $K \geq 2.5$ is given by the simple formula

$$C_a/C_b = [(K + 2)(K - 2)]^{-1/2}.$$

trol analytical errors within the laboratory, has been confirmed under practical quality control rules and turns out to be an appropriate standard for laboratory practice regardless of clinical opinion about medically significant changes.

Since both systematic bias and imprecision may increase the rate of false-positive decisions, total analytical error (TAE) must be shared between these two sources. Recently, Klee (1993) has remarked that, in order to have a reasonable chance of detecting unacceptable assay bias in the presence of imprecision through quality control rules, maximally allowable imprecision σ_a should be less than half the allowable bias B. Thus, for example, if the Cotlove limit is applied to the right-hand side of Equation (8.2), as suggested earlier, systematic bias should be $\leq 0.45\sigma_b$, while σ_a should be $\leq 0.22\sigma_b$. The square root of the sum of the squares will then be $\leq 0.5\sigma_b$.

This argument appears to run counter to our earlier finding that bias has a much greater effect than imprecision on the rate of false-positive decisions in diagnostic screening situations. Detailed discussion of modern quality control procedures for detecting analytical error in the clinical laboratory is outside the purview of this book, but this apparent conflict should be examined further.

8.3.2 Modeling by Fraser et al.

Fraser et al. (1990) used essentially the same basic model as Linnet although they assumed that with controlled conditions on tourniquet use, previous diet and exercise, etc., pre-analytical variations could be neglected. In addition, they left the probability level of false-positive decision with respect to the significance of an observed change open to the physician's discretion. In symbols, the critical change Δ_c may then be expressed as

$$\Delta_c > \sqrt{2}Z(C_a^2 + C_b^2)^{1/2} \qquad (8.7)$$

where Z, as usual, is the Normal deviate associated with a certain probability of false-positive decision that the change warrants some medical action, when in fact the true change is zero. Then,

$$C_a < [(\Delta_c^2/2Z^2) - C_b^2]^{1/2} \tag{8.8}$$

These authors pointed out that the vignettes in Skendzel et al.'s questionnaire for clinicians use such words as "convince," "indicate," "suggest," "lead one to believe," or "prompt" to describe the effect of a given numerical change on the clinician's belief that a medically significant change in the patient's condition has occurred. Now, Skendzel et al. (1985) used only one of these words or phrases in each vignette, but Fraser et al. consider that such words represent a graded response by the physician that could be applied to a single analyte in any one clinical situation. Specifically, a change that "convinces" the responding clinician would be larger, and therefore less likely to mislead, than a change that "indicates," which in turn would be larger than a change that simply "suggests." Of course, the larger the change, the higher the Z value associated with that change. If such changes can be identified in a given clinical condition, and appropriate Z values attached to them, then, assuming C_b is known, Equation (8.8) can be used to calculate the required analytical imprecision C_a.

Unfortunately, the arithmetic is likely to lead to different estimates of C_a for different specified critical changes. For practical purposes, one value of C_a would have to be selected. This might be the median or the smallest value. Another possibility is to begin by setting C_a at a fraction of C_b (e.g., one-half), then choose two operationally different Z values, calculate the corresponding values of Δ_c, and see whether these appear reasonable in terms of clinical practice. The presence of intermittent bias complicates this solution, however, and it would be more practical to accept a single action point used in clinical practice, attach a low probability of false-positive decision to this point, then preset C_a and evaluate the resulting limit of bias. In Section 8.5, we discuss a specific example of such calculations, the assay of glycolated hemoglobin HbA_{1c}, in monitoring diabetes mellitus (Larsen et al., 1991).

A consensus of medical opinion can be a valuable guide to the determination of analytical goals. As we have seen, when all sources of variability in observed results are taken into account, especially biological variation, such a consensus does not necessarily imply looser requirements than the current state of the art. On the contrary, widespread acceptance by physicians of new criteria for interpreting biochemical tests may well lead to more stringent goals for analytical accuracy. When, as in the case of cholesterol, the medical profession decides on the basis of epidemiological evidence that specific cutpoints should be used as reference values for interpreting a test result, then immediately a higher level of analytical accuracy is necessary than that heretofore considered adequate.

Moreover, as Linnet pointed out, and Westgard and Burnett (1990) have emphasized, analytical standards must be sufficient to maintain a consensus-based medically required level of accuracy during times of unstable operations within the laboratory as well as in normal circumstances when the analytical method is stable and working properly. If the maximally tolerable level of TAE to meet these clinical and laboratory specifications is beyond the reach of current methods, other steps may be taken: for example, preparing more than one specimen from a given blood sample and running analyses in replicate. This alternative would reduce within-run imprecision but not have much effect on long-term analytical imprecision. Securing additional blood samples at set intervals of time while the patient was in steady state would be a way of both reducing long-term analytical imprecision and overcoming within-subject biological variation. We discuss these possibilities further in the following section.

8.4 ANALYTICAL GOALS AROUND CUTPOINTS OF RISK

Requirements for analytical accuracy are most demanding when particular values of a biochemical test are designated by clinicians as medical decision points applicable to every individual. Selected cutpoints are used in diagnostic screening for a given disease; for example, the limits of the 95 percent reference range often serve this purpose. There is, however, a basic difference between the use of cutpoints in diagnostic screening and their use in the situation discussed in this section.

In screening, two overlapping distributions of test values are postulated, one referring to the population known to be harboring the disease, and the other to the population known to be free of the disease. Probabilities of false-positive decisions (1 minus the specificity of the test) and false-negative decisions (1 minus the sensitivity) are *averages* across these distributions of the (0,1) decision made in each individual case. In the present context, only one distribution of test values is supposed, that representing a population of individuals *at risk* of contracting the disease *at some time in the future*.

It is this concept of future risk rather than existing disease that distinguishes the two clinical situations. And it is this same concept that distinguishes the kind of epidemiological information on which reference values are based in each situation. In diagnostic screening, the information is retrospective, that is, from persons whose disease status is known. In the determination of risk cutpoints, the information is prospective. A body of individuals with certain initial characteristics, including the values of selected biochemical tests, is followed over time to find out who among them develop the disease in question. The probability of development of the disease is then plotted against initial value of the analyte, and from this graph biochemical decision points for medical action to help prevent future occurrence of the disease are determined.

Figure 1.1 illustrated such a graph taken from the Report of the National Cholesterol Education Program (NCEP) Expert Panel (1988). As noted in Chapter 1, the NCEP identified two cutpoints for serum cholesterol: 200 mg/dL (5.17 mmol/L) and 240 mg/dL (6.21 mmol/L). Values less than the first cutpoint were considered "desirable," values equal to or greater than the second cutpoint were considered high, and values of 200–239 mg/dL were classified as "borderline-high." Patients with borderline-high values but without definite CHD or two other risk factors for CHD were to be provided with information about low cholesterol diets and rechecked annually. Cutpoints were also set for LDL-cholesterol at two-thirds the corresponding values for total cholesterol.

Analytical goals for maximal allowable imprecision and bias in the determination of serum cholesterol were set by the Laboratory Standardization Panel (LSP) of the NCEP (1990) at interim values of ≤5 percent and "ideal" values of ≤3 percent to be achieved by 1992. To develop a statistical basis for such goals, we need to redefine the clinical sensitivity and specificity of a biochemical analyte in the context of a single continuous distribution of population values marked by specified cutpoints of risk.

In this context, sensitivity and specificity are defined at the level of the individual rather than as averages across a distribution of patients. Let μ_i represent the true value of the analyte in the ith patient at the time of sampling (neglecting pre-analytical variation), while x_i is the measured value and x_0 denotes a cutpoint, Then (Harris, 1979), the sensitivity of a measurement is equal to the probability that $x_i \geq x_0$, given that $\mu_i \geq x_0$, while the specificity is equal to the probability that $x_i < x_0$, given that $\mu_i < x_0$. Suppose that measured values are free of imprecision or bias and Normally distributed with standard deviation σ_{bi}, the biological variation within the ith patient. Then sensitivity and specificity are the same for a given numerical distance between μ_i and x_0 and may be written

$$\text{Sensitivity} = \text{specificity} = \int_{-\infty}^{z_{0i}} \phi\,(z)\,dz \qquad (8.9)$$

where

$$z_{0i} = [|\mu_i - x_0|]/\sigma_{bi}$$

Under error-free conditions, sensitivity and specificity are at a minimum of 50 percent when $\mu_i = x_0$ and approach 100 percent as the difference between these two quantities increases. Note again that sensitivity and specificity defined here are not average quantities as in diagnostic screening but vary from one individual to another depending on μ_i and σ_{bi}.

Relying largely on the work of Ross (1988) and Ross and Tholen (1987), the LSP proposed a goal for total analytical error in the determination of cholesterol such that the "diagnostic efficiency" (DE) of a measurement in the absence of analytical error would be degraded no more than 10 percent by the presence of bias and imprecision. DE was defined as equivalent to the term "efficiency," coined by Galen and Gambino (1975, p. 33) to denote the weighted average of sensitivity and specificity in the usual context of diagnostic screening, where the weight is the prevalence of the disease. For consistency with the LSP report and Ross (1988), we assume a prevalence of 50 percent (i.e., equal weighting).[8]

Simulation studies by Ross (1988) indicated that the effect of analytical error on DE was maximal for values of μ_i such that $|\mu_i - x_0| = 0.94\sigma_{bi}$. In addition to a maximal loss of 10 percent DE under these conditions, the LSP also recommended that no more than 5 percent of DE should be lost through analytical error when $|\mu_i - x_0| = 2\sigma_{bi}$. To illustrate the effects of these recommendations, let us calculate DE for such individuals in the absence of analytical error ($B = k = 0$) and with both bias and imprecision (C_a) set at 5 percent and then at 3 percent of the cutpoint value of 240 mg/dL cholesterol, as recommended by the LSP.

Suppose the ith patient exhibits average biological variation in cholesterol, that is, $C_{bi} = C_b = 5.4$ percent (see Table 8.1), or $\sigma_b = 12.96$ ml/dL at $x_0 = 240$ mg/dL. Suppose further that $|\mu_i - x_0| = 0.94\sigma_b = 12$ mg/dL (i.e., $\mu_i = 228$ or 252

---

[8] This is certainly not realistic. On the other hand, an extended definition of efficiency could define the weight to represent a combination of prevalence and the relative importance assigned to sensitivity as opposed to specificity. In the context of screening for risk of coronary heart disease, such a combined weight might well be close to one-half.

mg/dL). From Equation (8.9), the error-free DE for this patient equals 82 percent. For another patient with $|\mu_j - x_0| = 2\sigma_b = 26$ mg/dL, error-free DE equals 97.8 percent. The effect of imprecision is to reduce both sensitivity and specificity by the same amount. On the other hand, positive bias increases sensitivity but decreases specificity, while negative bias has the reverse effect. However, giving equal weight to both sensitivity and specificity, the effect on DE is the same regardless of the direction of bias.

Now, whatever goal is set for σ_a, it will represent some multiple k_i of the ith patient's biological variation σ_{bi}. If, in addition, a maximal bias $|B|$ mg/dL is allowed, then Equation (8.9) holds with $z_{0i} = [|\mu_i - x_0| \pm |B|]/[\sigma_{bi}(1 + k_i^2)^{1/2}]$, where $|B|$ is added to compute sensitivity and subtracted to compute specificity. Consider limits on σ_a and B set at 5 percent of 240, or 12 mg/dL. Then, for $\sigma_{bi} = \sigma_b = 12.96$ mg/dL, and $|\mu_i - x_0| = 12$ mg/dL, $k_i = 12/12.96 = 0.93$, and $z_{0i} = (12 \pm 12)/[12.96 (1 + .93^2)^{1/2}]$. Sensitivity is increased to 0.912, specificity reduced to 0.50, and DE degraded to 70.6 percent, a decline of 13.9 percent from the error-free value of 82 percent in this patient. In the jth patient, for whom biological variation is the same but $|\mu_j - x_0| = 26$ mg/dL, DE is degraded to 88.5 percent, a loss of 9.5 percent from the error-free value of 97.8 percent. Neither of these results satisfy the goals of the LSP with respect to limits on the maximal loss of diagnostic efficiency in a patient.

Under the more stringent analytical goals of 3 percent bias and imprecision, the same calculations show that DE is reduced to 76.5 percent at $|\mu_i - x_0| = 12$ mg/dL, a loss of 6.7 percent. At $|\mu_j - x_0| = 26$ mg/dL, efficiency is 94.2 percent, a loss of 3.7 percent. Therefore, these analytical goals do meet the requirements of the LSP.

The preceding calculations used 5.4 percent as the average within-subject biological CV (C_b) of total cholesterol, as in the LSP report. A recent detailed meta-analysis of past studies by Smith et al. (1993) estimated C_b at 6.1 percent. Using this estimate produces a slight decrease in the percentage losses of DE computed above, but does not change the conclusion that allowing bias and imprecision as high as 5 percent does not meet the stated requirements of the LSP whereas an upper limit of 3 percent clearly does meet these requirements.

However, the LSP report (p. 36) sets an additional requirement on the measurement of total cholesterol in the ith person, namely, that total variation, $C_{ti} = (C_{bi}^2 + C_a^2 + B^2)^{1/2}$, should not exceed 5 percent, so that a confidence interval of width 10 percent about a single test value would have 95 percent probability of containing the true mean μ_i. Even with C_a and B no higher than 3 percent, and $C_{bi} = C_b = 6.1$ percent, this limit on C_{ti} cannot be met with only one measurement. Therefore, the LSP recommends that at this level of analytical error, two specimens be obtained at least 1 week apart but within a period of two months, and the results averaged.[9] This would reduce C_{bi}^2 and C_a^2 by a factor of 2, and, in the absence of systematic bias, would reduce C_{ti} to less than 5 percent.

A further difficulty arises because many individuals exhibit biological variability greater than the average value. Cooper et al. (1992, 1994) estimate that C_{bi} may range up to 10.9 percent. These authors propose that two to five specimens be collected during a 2-month period, the number depending on the range of results as each new value is obtained. They provide (1994) a table of upper limits of the relative range (range divided by the mean of the first two specimens) for guidance to the clinician in deciding whether or not to seek an additional specimen before estimating the patient's true cholesterol level.

Finally, Westgard et al. (1991) examine various goals for bias and imprecision against a variety of single and multi-rule quality control procedures under unstable laboratory operations. They employ a model based on the cutpoints for total cholesterol recommended by the NCEP that is essentially another definition of DE although different from that proposed

---

[9] Rotterdam et al. (1987) had shown that a time interval of at least 4 days between specimens is required to allow within-subject biological variation to reach a plateau.

by Ross (1988). Specifically, they require that (1) the probability that the laboratory will report a test value $x_i \geq 240$ mg/dL in a patient for whom $\mu_i \leq 200$ mg/dL is ≤ 0.05, and (2) the probability that $x_i \leq 200$ mg/dL when $\mu_i \geq 240$ mg/dL is also ≤ 0.05. The first requirement represents a definition of specificity; the second, a definition of sensitivity. Both are required to equal or exceed 0.95. Using Equation (8.9), we can test to see whether bias and imprecision of no more than 3 percent will satisfy these requirements, assuming stable laboratory operations. For $|\mu_i - x_0| = 40$ mg/dL, $\sigma_{bi} = 6.1$ percent (Westgard et al. use 6.5 percent) and bias and imprecision of 3 percent, sensitivity is 99.8 percent and specificity, 97.8 percent. The percentages are reversed when the bias is negative. Therefore, the specifications set by Westgard et al. are satisfied at these levels of analytical error when laboratory operations are stable.

When they are unstable, as in the presence of a transient systematic error above the allowable bias, Westgard et al. show that these levels of bias and imprecision will not be adequate to allow detection of the out-of-control condition with 90 percent probability at a false rejection level (Type I error) ≤ 0.1 under either single or multi-rule control procedures with up to four control measurements. However, if two specimens are collected from the patient over the time span mentioned above, reducing analytical precision and within-subject biological variation but not bias, then the (single-sample) limits of 3 percent would be sufficient to allow detection of out-of-control systematic error under all current quality control procedures using four control measurements at false rejection levels around 0.05. These results confirm the recommendations of the LSP that two serial specimens should be obtained from each patient and the results averaged. They are also consistent with the recommendations of Cooper et al. noted earlier for additional specimens when the patient exhibits above-average biological variability. Imprecision of ≤ 3 percent in the measurement of total cholesterol satisfies the rule of Cotlove et al. (assuming $\sigma_b \geq 6.1$ percent) and would continue to do so if results for two serial specimens were averaged.

8.5 EXAMPLE

Glycated hemoglobin HbA_{1c} is one of a series of compounds formed from the reaction between glucose and hemoglobin. It has been shown (see Larsen et al., 1990, for further references) to be a good index for use in monitoring metabolic control in diabetics. Recently, Larsen et al. (1991) have examined several different strategies for developing allowable goals for analytical error in measuring this compound. These different approaches represent the general methods discussed in the two preceding sections.

Since no accepted reference method was available, an "absolute" measure of bias could not be obtained. Initial studies and literature review by Larsen et al. (1990) selected the method of isoelectric focusing as highly specific for HbA_{1c}. The superior performance of this method was confirmed by recovery and linearity studies. The unit of measurement of HbA_{1c} is as a percentage of total hemoglobin in red blood cells.

In place of bias, the authors define systematic error (SE) as a measure of transient shift that may arise under stable laboratory operations in the interim between two serial measurements of the analyte. This adds a bit of semantic confusion because earlier we mentioned that such shifts were usually included in the definition of long-term analytical imprecision. Besides, the symbol SE was employed by Linnet and Westgard et al. to denote a shift indicative of unstable laboratory operations. Here, Larsen et al. appear to be using SE in essentially the same sense as Linnet and Westgard et al., but do not raise the issue of whether their estimates of maximal tolerable SE under various goal-setting strategies are likely to be detected under one or another quality control procedure.

The basic model postulates a critical change Δ_c between two serial measurements expressible in terms of analytical imprecision, average within-subject biological variation, and SE, as follows,

$$\Delta_c = \sqrt{2}Z(C_a^2 + C_b^2)^{1/2} + SE \qquad (8.10)$$

Setting the probability of a false-positive decision on the medical significance of the observed change to its usual (two-sided) value of 0.05, $\sqrt{2}Z = 2.77$. Estimates of C_b came from a study of 30 patients with insulin-dependent diabetes mellitus in apparently steady-state metabolic control who had been followed in the outpatient clinic for over a year with repeated measurements of HbA_{1c}. In fact, the patients appear to have divided into three groups who reached different but very stable levels of HbA_{1c} (8, 10, and 12 percent). These were taken as reflecting good, fair, and poor metabolic control, respectively. Estimated values of σ_b within each group were 0.70, 0.41, and 0.65 percent HbA_{1c}, respectively. Using the value 0.41, corresponding to $C_b = 4.1$ percent, the following strategies were considered to determine goals for C_a and SE:

1. With $\sqrt{2}Z = 2.77$, set $C_a = \frac{1}{2}C_b = 2.1$ percent when SE $= 0$ (the Cotlove et al. rule), and solve Equation (8.10) for $\Delta_c = 12.8$ percent, or 1.3 percent HbA_{1c}. Using this value as the maximal allowable observed change when the true value is zero, combinations of C_a and SE that satisfy this limit may be computed and plotted as curve 1 in Figure 8.4. At $C_a = 0$, SE $= 1.44$ percent, or 0.14 percent HbA_{1c}.

2a. A change of 1.0 percent HbA_{1c} "calls attention" to a possible minor change in the patient's condition. Larsen et al. associated this with the Normal deviate 1.28 (two-sided probability of false-positive decision equal to 20 percent). Under this strategy, the medically significant change Δ_c is predetermined at 10 percent of the mean. Inserting this value into Equation (8.10) along with $Z = 1.28$, then $C_a = 3.7$ percent of the mean HbA_{1c}, when SE $= 0$, while SE $= 2.6$ percent of the mean when $C_a = 0$. These and other combinations are plotted on curve 2a in Figure 8.4.

2b) An increase of 2.0 percent HbA_{1c} (20 percent of the mean) induces medical intervention. The authors associate this action with the Normal deviate 2.58, a two-sided probability of false-positive decision equal to 1 percent. Using these values in Equation (8.10), $C_a = 3.7$ percent when SE $= 0$, and SE $=$

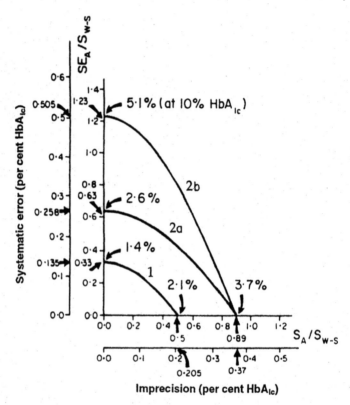

Fig. 8.4 Analytical goals for imprecision and bias according to three different strategies for medical action: (1), (2a), and (2b); see text for details. (From Larsen et al., 1991, with permission.)

5.1 percent when $C_a = 0$. These and other combinations are plotted on Curve 2b in Figure 8.4.

Clearly, the three curves do not lead to common estimates of allowable limits of analytical precision or systematic error, illustrating the difficulty (some might say futility) of trying to translate such state-of-mind descriptors as "convincing" or "indicating" to specific probabilities that would yield consistent estimates of maximal allowable analytical error. An alternative strategy would be to preset C_a and SE (or bias when a reference method is available) at a specified fraction (or separate fractions) of C_b, solve for Δ_c at one (or more) probability levels, and evaluate the results in terms of clinical practice.

It would seem more practical, on the other hand, to use the action level currently recognized by clinicians, 2.0 percent HbA_{1c}, assign to it a very low probability of false-positive decision (say, 0.5 percent, or $Z = 2.58$ in accordance with Larsen et al.), set $C_a = \frac{1}{2}C_b$, and solve Equation (8.10) for SE. Under these conditions, the maximal allowable SE = 3.2 percent of the mean HbA_{1c}.

Finally, Larsen et al. introduce a medically determined cut-point in the manner of the NCEP recommendations for cholesterol. In this case, however, there seems to be some disagreement in the literature as to whether the best value for x_0 is 7.5 or 9.0 percent HbA_{1c}. Selecting the lower value, the authors employ essentially the criterion of Ross (1988), adopted by the Laboratory Standardization Panel of the NCEP, namely, that analytical imprecision and bias should not degrade diagnostic efficiency by more than 10 percent. As noted in Section 8.4, Ross found that the effect of analytical error on diagnostic efficiency was greatest when $|\mu_i - x_0| = 0.94\sigma_{bi}$. Assuming C_{bi} is at the average level of 4.1 percent, $\sigma_{bi} = 0.31$ percent HbA_{1c} at $x_0 = 7.5$ percent, so that we focus attention on parameter values μ_i, σ_{bi} such that $|\mu_i - x_0| = 0.94\sigma_{bi} = 0.29$ percent HbA_{1c}, where DE is 82 percent in the absence of analytical error.

Setting both imprecision and SE at 3 percent ($\times 7.5 = 0.225$ percent HbA_{1c}), then $k_i = 0.225/0.31 = 0.73$. Repeating the earlier calculations for cholesterol [Equation (8.9) with z_{0i} adjusted for bias and imprecision), we find that sensitivity when $|\mu_i - x_0| = 0.29$ percent HbA_{1c} is increased to 0.910, specificity is decreased to 0.567, and DE is reduced to 73.9 percent, giving equal weighting to false-positive and false-negative diagnoses. This represents a loss of 9.9 percent from error-free DE, just within the Ross criterion.

If $|\mu_j - x_0| = 2\sigma_b$, or 0.62, calculations show that 3 percent imprecision and bias degrade DE by 6.2 percent, slightly higher than Ross's criterion of 5 percent. To assure a high probability of detecting unstable laboratory operations through reasonable quality control rules, as advised by Linnet and Westgard et al. (Sections 8.3 and 8.4), the ideal goals for imprecision and bias should probably be reduced to no more than 2 percent.

8.6   REMARKS

As indicated above, the last few years have seen a flurry of publications on the subject of analytical goals for clinical laboratories. Studies of clinical opinion concerning medically significant changes in biochemical test results have been undertaken, mathematical models relating such changes to allowable limits for analytical error have been developed, and the power of quality control procedures to detect transient inaccuracies beyond these limits has been investigated.

At the same time, in at least one clinical condition, coronary heart disease, epidemiological evidence of future risk of disease relative to current test values for certain analytes has led to general agreement among clinicians on appropriate cutpoints for medical action. Such cutpoints may be entirely unrelated to the 95 percent reference limits in the general population.

All of these activities will undoubtedly continue and may become more complex as new kinds of biochemical analytes replace those in current use or multiple disease conditions are associated with changes in a given analyte. In the next chapter, we extend the search for analytical goals to a relatively recent, but increasingly important, area of clinical laboratory operations: therapeutic drug monitoring.

9

ANALYTICAL GOALS IN THERAPEUTIC DRUG MONITORING

9.1 INTRODUCTION

The assay of serum or plasma for therapeutic drugs is a relative newcomer to routine clinical laboratory operations, starting in the early 1970s (Marks, 1985). Research studies have shown that responses to drugs are more closely correlated with blood concentration than with dose [a review of this literature has been provided by Burton et al. (1985)]. Clinical experience has demonstrated the importance of individualizing drug therapy because of wide patient-to-patient variation in the parameters of drug absorption, distribution, and elimination as well as in physiological response.

These conditions indicate the need for patient monitoring of therapeutic drugs through laboratory assay of blood specimens. However, as specialists in this field have made clear (e.g., Hallworth, 1988; Schumacher and Barr, 1989), an accurate determination of drug concentration in blood will not improve patient care unless the general pharmacokinetics of that particular drug in the body are understood, the individual response characteristics of the patient are appreciated, and important pre-analytical conditions (such as the elapsed time between adminstration of the dose and blood drawing) have been met.

Contributions to the development and application of computerized statistical methods for individualizing drug therapy have been made over the past 25 years by Sheiner and colleagues (e.g., Sheiner et al., 1972, 1977, 1979b, recently reviewed in Sheiner and Ludden, 1992). We also note the closely related work of Kelman et al. (1982), and valuable review articles in this area by Vožeh and Steimer (1985) and Whiting et al. (1986). These methods, now applied to many therapeutic drugs, are based on Bayesian forecasting techniques in which a prior multivariate Normal distribution of pharmacokinetic parameters with known means and among-patients variances is modified by one or two assays in the patient to produce estimates of the individual's parameters. These are then fed back into an appropriate pharmacokinetic mathematical model to obtain estimates of required dosages and expected future blood levels.

Fundamental to the proper administration of drug therapy and interpretation of blood concentrations is the *therapeutic range*. This is defined as the range between the minimum effective concentration of a given drug in the serum or plasma and the maximum safe (nontoxic) concentration. The therapeutic range is somewhat analogous to the reference range for an endogenous blood constituent such as cholesterol or glucose. That is, the therapeutic range reflects within- and among-patients variation with respect to the (physiologically) best concentration for eliciting the desired response while avoiding dangerous side effects. On the other hand, the therapeutic range cannot ethically be determined by exposing a large sample of healthy reference humans to a range of doses of a drug supposed to alleviate a specific pathological condition.

Investigation of a therapeutic drug requires, first, dosage–response studies in animals to reveal the nature of any toxic effects that may be anticipated in humans. A recent review by Voisin et al. (1990) discusses methods used to extrapolate animal toxicity to humans. In the earlier days of therapeutic drug monitoring (TDM), animal toxicity studies were accompanied by retrospective examination of the responses of patients, and their blood concentrations, to prescribed dosages. Today, if animal or in vitro pharmacology studies indicate that a new drug is worth further investigation, randomized controlled (or concentration-controlled) clinical trials (e.g., Sanathanan and Peck, 1991) must be undertaken in human volunteers.

For many drugs, the therapeutic range is quite narrow. Therefore, the primary goal of TDM is to achieve as soon as possible, and maintain, the best dosage and blood concentration for the individual patient. Knowledge of a suitable pharmacokinetic model for the drug and the general distribution of pharmacokinetic parameters is a necessary step in reaching this goal. These parameters are known to vary substantially by age, state of renal function, and other characteristics of the patient.

This chapter is limited to the subject of analytical goals in TDM. The past two decades have seen a continued improvement in the analytical specificity and accuracy of drug measurement procedures. The most precise and generally satisfactory methods in common use today for routine TDM appear to be homogeneous immunoassay. The literature on analytical goals in TDM is still very sparse. For example, TDM was not included among the subjects discussed at the symposium on analytical goals and medical relevance (1993) sponsored by the American Association for Clinical Chemistry. In the following section, we examine certain methods that have been proposed to date for arriving at analytical goals.

The drug theophylline serves as a useful example for specific applications because it has a narrow therapeutic range and follows a relatively simple pharmacokinetic model within the body. In addition, recent literature contains data on patient-to-patient and within-patient variability in theophylline levels in blood. General information about its therapeutic use and monitoring may be found, for example, in a review by Hendeles and Weinberger (1981). Theophylline has been used for many years as a bronchodilator (relaxing bronchial smooth muscle) in treating acute and chronic asthma. In acute attacks, the drug is administered intravenously, followed by oral dosage to prevent the symptoms of chronic asthma. Its therapeutic range is 10–20 mg/L with toxic reactions likely to occur when the blood concentration exceeds 25 mg/L. However, these values are lower for neonates and children. Metabolism and elimination from the body (clearance) occur at a rate relatively high in neonates and gradually decreasing with age.

9.2 MODELS FOR ANALYTICAL GOALS IN TDM

9.2.1 Fraser's Model

To our knowledge, the first attempt to develop a statistical model for determining analytical goals in TDM was published only recently by Fraser (1987). Fraser makes use of a particularly simple mathematical relationship between the theoretical maximum and minimum concentrations of a drug after repeated intravenous dosing at fixed intervals of time. Under such circumstances, the concentration–time curve after a single dose follows the simple exponential form:

$$C(t) = C(0) e^{-k_e t}, \tag{9.1}$$

where the initial concentration $C(0)$ equals D/V, the amount of dose divided by the volume of the vascular compartment, and k_e is the rate of elimination of the drug from the blood.

After repeated dosing over several half-lives of the drug, the blood concentration rises to a steady state such that each new dose produces a maximum and minimum concentration during that dosing interval. These concentrations are given by the formulas (e.g., Welling, 1986, p. 190),

$$C_{ss}(max) = D[V(1 - e^{-k_e \tau})]^{-1},$$
$$C_{ss}(min) = De^{-k_e \tau} [V(1 - e^{-k_e \tau})]^{-1}, \tag{9.2}$$

where τ is the (constant) interval between doses. Then the ratio $R = C_{ss}(max)/C_{ss}(min) = e^{k_e \tau}$. The half-life of the drug, the time at which $C(t)$ in Equation (9.1) equals $\frac{1}{2}C(0)$, is given by $t_{1/2} = (\ln 2)/k_e$. Therefore, $R = 2^{\tau/t_{1/2}}$, a function of dose interval and half-life.

Fraser considers the difference $C_{ss}(max) - C_{ss}(min)$ as representing a subject-specific 95 percent reference range with length equal to four times the average within-patient biological standard deviation of serum measurements. Then he invokes the Cotlove et al. rule that analytical imprecision should not exceed half the average within-person biological variation. In terms of coefficient of variation (CV), this becomes

$$CV_a \le \tfrac{1}{2}CV_b = \tfrac{1}{2}\sigma_b/\mu. \tag{9.3}$$

Fraser takes μ as $\frac{1}{2}[C_{ss}(max) + C_{ss}(min)]$, so that (9.3) becomes

$$CV_a \le \tfrac{1}{4}[C_{ss}(max) - C_{ss}(min)]/[C_{ss}(max) + C_{ss}(min)] \tag{9.4}$$

Introducing the ratio $R = C_{ss}(max)/C_{ss}(min) = 2^{\tau/t_{1/2}}$,

$$C_a \leq \tfrac{1}{4}[2^{\tau/t_{1/2}} - 1]/[2^{\tau/t_{1/2}} + 1] \times 100 \text{ percent.} \qquad (9.5)$$

As the ratio of dose interval to half-life $(\tau/t_{1/2})$ increases, this expression for C_a increases to 25 percent. Therefore, if $\tau/t_{1/2}$ varies for different population groups, one should choose the lowest value, leading to the most stringent analytical goal. In children, the half-life of theophylline (about 4 hr) is about half that in nonsmoking adults, but the dosing interval (typically $\leq$ 6 hr) is usually less than half that in adults. If $\tau/t_{1/2}$ is taken equal to 6/4, or 1.5, then, using Equation (9.5), C_a should not exceed 12 percent, a figure that Fraser accepts as satisfactory.

In our opinion, Fraser's model suffers a serious conceptual flaw in treating the difference $C_{ss}(max) - C_{ss}(min)$ as a statistical quantity, a 95 percent reference range arising from within-patient biological variability. This difference is in fact a purely deterministic expression from a mathematical pharmacokinetic model. To represent it as a portion of a statistical distribution is not valid, in our view.

Moreover, even if one could justify this representation, the model pertains only to intravenous drug administration. The pharmacokinetics of drugs taken orally is considerably more complicated, involving absorption from the gut into the blood. The effect of repeated oral dosing is to reduce $C_{ss}(max)$ and increase $C_{ss}(min)$ while leaving the sum of these quantities unchanged (e.g., Welling, 1986, p. 197). Under Fraser's model, this would imply a goal of smaller analytical imprecision than required for assaying serum concentrations following intravenous administration of drug. It may be that analytical imprecision, even as percentage variation, depends on pharmacokinetic parameters such as half-life or clearance since these affect the mean steady-state concentration. However, it does not seem reasonable that assay imprecision should be related to whether the drug is given intravenously or orally when the mean steady-state concentration is the same in both cases.

Fraser and Lipworth (1988) noted that in two earlier studies (Halkin et al., 1982, and Taylor et al., 1984) average biological CV's in steady-state theophylline concentrations over periods of 4–7 days following slow-release dosages ranged from 17.9 to 22.7 percent, averaging 20.6 percent.[1] An analytical goal of less than 12 percent imprecision calculated by Fraser thus slightly exceeds the criterion recommended by Cotlove et al.(Chapter 8) The analytical CV's reported by Taylor et al. and Halkin et al. were 6.4 percent and 14.5 percent, respectively, the latter representing combined within- and between-run imprecision. High-performance liquid chromatography (HPLC) was used in both studies.

---

[1] Since data on within-subject biological variation from the study of Halkin et al. (1982) are referred to by both Fraser and Lipworth and by Jenny (1991) and are used in our calculations, some details of this study should be noted. Halkin et al. studied fifteen adult chronic asthmatic patients sampled on 6 consecutive days after a week of treatment with slow-release theophylline. Prior to the use of the slow-release formulation, patients had received ordinary theophylline sodium glycinate tablets for a period of 2 weeks, and were in remission with theophylline levels in steady state. Slow-release capsules were administered at 12-hour intervals. Blood specimens were obtained at 1 and 5 hours after the morning dose.

Halkin et al. (Table 2) listed within-patient CV's of both the 1-hour and 5-hour specimens. Average CV's were 24.3 and 21.8 percent, respectively. We have used the average of these results, 23 percent. The authors reported analytical CV's averaging 2.5 percent (within-run) and 14.3 percent (between-run), giving an estimated long-term analytical CV of 14.5 percent. Therefore, we estimated average within-patient biological variation to be $(23^2 - 14.5^2)^{1/2}$, or 17.8 percent, somewhat less than the figure given by Fraser and Lipworth for this study. Jenny cites the study by Halkin et al. as reporting 5.8 percent for this quantity, but we cannot find evidence in their report for this extremely small value.

9.2.2 Jenny's Models

Jenny (1991) proposed two possible ways of calculating goals for the precision of drug assays in blood. The first of these used the procedure suggested by Harris (1979), represented by Equation (8.9), intended for use when a specific cutpoint for risk has been determined. In TDM, the upper limit of the therapeutic range defines such a cutpoint. Jenny sets a criterion for analytical error such that diagnostic efficiency (DE, see Section 8.4) at this cutpoint will not be degraded more than 5 percent beyond that found in the absence of such error. Both Jenny and Fraser argue that the systematic bias of a truly satisfactory assay procedure for TDM must be zero; that is, the assay must be specific for the drug in original form, free of interference effects from metabolites. Random biases are included in the definition of between-run imprecision, as mentioned earlier. Under this condition, either sensitivity or specificity represents DE and may be calculated from Equation (8.9).

Jenny applied this methodology to determination of an analytical goal for measurement of theophylline (therapeutic range, 10–20 mg/L). Setting the individual's biological variation CV_{bi} equal to the average value $CV_b = 17.8$ percent (our estimate, see footnote 1) and $x_o = 20$ mg/L, σ_b at this concentration equals 3.6 mg/L. For $|\mu_i - x_0| = 0.94\,\sigma_b$ (the point at which the percentage effect of analytical imprecision on DE is maximal), we find, as before, that DE = 82 percent. To decrease this by no more than 5 percent, that is, to no less than 78 percent, we set $z_0 = 0.94/(1 + k^2)^{1/2} = 0.772$, and solve for $k = 0.69$. In other words, maximal acceptable imprecision in the assay of serum theophylline would be 0.69 × 17.8, or 12.5 percent. This figure is remarkably close to the goal estimated by Fraser from a deterministic model of intravenous dosing with selected values for dosing interval and half-life. It is slightly less than the long-term analytical CV reported by Halkin et al.

The second method discussed by Jenny for determining analytical goals in TDM assays is based on a well-known empirical formula published by Chiou et al. (1978) for estimating drug clearance (Cl) during constant-rate intravenous infusion. It is based on the standard one-compartment model for intravenous dosing, requires two successive measurements of blood concentration, and is intended for use in individualizing blood therapy. By estimating the patient's clearance, the proper infusion rate to achieve a desired steady-state concentration may be quickly estimated. The Chiou formula may be written

$$\text{Cl} = \frac{2R_0}{C_1 + C_2} + \frac{2V(C_1 - C_2)}{(C_1 + C_2)(t_2 - t_1)} \tag{9.6}$$

where R_0 denotes initial infusion rate, V, apparent volume of distribution, and C_1, C_2, the plasma concentrations measured at times t_1 and t_2 during the infusion process. The first specimen should be drawn about 5 hours after the beginning of infusion. Good agreement has been reported between clearances estimated from the Chiou formula and from Bayesian feedback programs (Manzanares et al., 1991; Sheiner and Beal, 1982). Multiplying the estimated clearance by the desired steady-state concentration C_{ss} provides an estimate of the appropriate infusion rate that may require modification of the initial rate to suit the individual patient.[2]

Jenny employs the propagation-of-error technique for relating the variance of Cl to the analytical variances of the measured concentrations. Assuming that the analytical errors in the two measurements are independent, this method provides an approximate formula for the variance of Cl in the form

---

[2] Assuming that C_{ss} is the mean steady-state concentration, multiplying by Cl estimated from intravenous drug dosing would also provide an estimate of oral dosage when the intravenous route for acute treatment is replaced by the oral route for chronic treatment. However, the dosage would then have to be divided by a fraction representing the "bioavailability" of the drug (i.e., that fraction of the oral dosage that is absorbed from the gut into the blood).

$$\text{Var Cl} = (\partial Cl/\partial C_1)^2 \,(\text{Var } C_1) + (\partial Cl/\partial C_2)^2(\text{Var } C_2),$$

$$(9.7)$$

where the partial derivatives are evaluated at the expected values of the variables, i.e., $E(C_1) = E(C_2) = C_{ss}$, the mean steady-state concentration. Taking $\text{Var } C_1 = \text{Var } C_2 = \text{Var } C$, we obtain

$$\text{Var Cl} = \left[\frac{R_0^2}{2C_{ss}^4} + \frac{2V^2}{C_{ss}^2 \,(t_2 - t_1)^2} \right] \text{Var } C \qquad (9.8)$$

The bracketed term on the right can be expressed entirely in terms of Cl (the true clearance of the drug in the given patient) and C_{ss} by noting (1) that $E(R_0) = C_{ss}\,Cl$; (2) that the interval $(t_2 - t_1)$ is some multiple, say k, of the drug's half-life $t_{1/2}$; and (3) that $t_{1/2}$ equals $0.693\,V/Cl$. With these substitutions, Equation (9.8) reduces to

$$[CV(Cl)]^2 = [(4.16/k^2) + 0.5]\,[CV(C)]^2 \qquad (9.9)$$

Now, following Jenny's lead,[3] we desire to estimate a new infusion rate (or oral dosage) for this patient such that the resulting steady-state mean concentration will, with 95 percent probability, lie within the therapeutic range of the drug. For theophylline, the width of this range is 10 mg/L. Since $C_{ss} = R/Cl$, this implies that the estimated infusion rate divided by the true clearance Cl should equal a target value of $C_{ss} = 15$ mg/L, while the 95 percent confidence interval $R_U - R_L = 4\sigma_R = 4(15)\sigma_{Cl}$, divided by Cl, should not exceed 10 mg/L. In other words, CV(Cl) should not exceed 10/60, or 16.6 percent.

It remains to set the time interval between the two specimen collections as a ratio of the half-life of the drug. Chiou et al. found from patient studies that good estimates of clearance were obtained for intervals of 1–3 half-lives, but did not rule

---

[3] The development following Equation (9.7) to this point is our own, not found in Jenny's paper.

out intervals of 30–50 percent of half-life. However, D'Argenio and Khakmahd (1983) concluded from computer simulation studies of theophylline that clinically significant estimation errors occur if the interval is less than one half-life. Setting $k = 1$, Equation (9.9) indicates that CV(C), the analytical goal for imprecision in assaying theophylline, should not exceed (16.6/2.16), or 7 percent. Values of $k > 1$ would produce larger values for CV(C), i.e., more lenient goals.

Clearly, this goal is considerably more stringent than that obtained from the earlier calculations involving reductions in diagnostic efficiency. Chiou et al. suggest even more precise measurement with analytical error not to exceed 5–6 percent. Such precision would be justified by the need to individualize therapy. It is attainable with present methods if the two blood specimens required in the Chiou formula are analyzed within the same run to avoid random biases. The analytical goal of 12.5 percent, based on biological variation and the therapeutic limit, is intended for general day-to-day monitoring of the patient and must allow for between-run analytical error. Thus, the two goals can coexist if the different purposes of results are recognized.

The model of Chiou et al. is based on the assumption that the pharmacokinetics of a drug following intravenous infusion can be reasonably well approximated by a linear one-compartment model. In contrast, Equation (8.9) may be thought of as an entirely statistical (i.e., nondeterministic) approach. Its advantage lies in its applicability to any therapeutic drug for which (1) the therapeutic range has been determined, and (2) average within-patient day-to-day biological variation around a steady-state concentration has been estimated.

10

REFERENCE VALUES IN THE FUTURE

10.1 INTRODUCTION

Relatively few changes have occurred over the past 20 years in the way reference values are applied to mainstream health care. We have, however, referred to several recent currents, statistical and clinical, that have already begun to affect the very definition as well as the clinical use of reference values. These include, for example, the selection of reference cutpoints based on prospective epidemiological studies of disease outcome. In Sections 1.7 and 8.4, we discussed such cutpoints in serum cholesterol, used now to indicate risk for the onset of coronary heart disease. Another important movement is toward the greater use of serial measurements and, consequently, person-specific reference values, in following healthy subjects and in patient management after treatment. Statistical methods in these contexts were the subject of Chapter 7. In addition, age-dependent centile curves of reference values, discussed in Chapter 5, will undoubtedly become more widely applied in clinical practice.

At this writing, rapid advances in medical information technology, laboratory automation, and molecular genetics, as well as increased concern for cost control, are producing changes in health care that will become even more dramatic in years to come. Each of these forces will affect medical practice as a whole, including the role of the clinical laboratory. Reference values, as tools in the interpretation of laboratory results, are likely to be influenced by fundamental changes in the practice of laboratory medicine within the entire field of health care. We will try in this final chapter to describe the effects of these modern advances on the practice of laboratory medicine, forecasting as best we can their likely effects on the definition and use of reference values. We start with the electronic medical record.

10.2 ELECTRONIC MEDICAL RECORD

The multiple provider and institutional environments characteristic of health care in the United States and the associated diverse patterns of care have resulted in a fragmented patient medical record. No single authority, whether it be health care provider (e.g., nurse or physician), institution (e.g., hospital or nursing home), or third-party payer (state or private insurance company) has responsibility for maintaining a comprehensive medical record. As a result, computerized information systems have been organized to support the ad hoc financial, administrative, and communication needs of individual institutions. The need for improved management of medical information through an integrated computer-based patient record system has received official recognition in a recent report by the Institute of Medicine of the National Academy of Science (Dick and Steen, 1991). Although there are still problems of standards development and funding (Barnett et al., 1993), and evolution of an optimal model on which to base such record systems (Essin, 1993; Frisse et al., 1994), the accelerating pace of change in health care is certain to dictate the ultimate development of an integrated computer-based patient record.

Standards for communicating information from one computerized system (e.g., the clinical laboratory) to another are critically needed. The earliest published standard came from a subcommittee of the American Society for Testing and Materials (ASTM) dealing primarily with the transfer of laboratory results from automated clinical laboratory instruments to laboratory information systems. New documents have been developed under the auspices of Health Level Seven (HL7), a consortium of vendors, hospitals and consultants to define standards for transmitting other information, such as billing, admission–discharge–transfer and physicians' orders within a hospital network of computers. In collaboration with ASTM, HL7 has defined a standard protocol to be used in communicating laboratory data in an electronic format. A sample communication in HL7 format is displayed in Figure 10.1. Various patient-identifying records, laboratory order records, and test results are shown. Reference values are among the items included in the test result record. The standard requires that all information be transmitted as printable characters. Individual items of information such as a patient's name or a test identifier are set off by unique delimiting characters.

Codifying laboratory information in a standardized form following the HL7 protocol will allow test results for the same patient to be collated from several laboratories into a single regional (or eventually, national) computer data base. Currently, networks of hospitals are rapidly forming to remain competitive under the managed care model for providing health care. As these hospital networks evolve, there will be strong motivation to integrate the computer-based medical information systems that serve them. Therefore, we can expect the formation of large health care computer networks in the near future. These networks will operate at least at the regional level and perhaps also at the national level.

10.2.1 Effects on Reference Values

The formation of a computer data base containing medical records that cover the patient's entire life, including laboratory data from virtually all the health care institutions that have provided him or her with care, opens up new opportunities and challenges for the appropriate use of reference values. For example, the effects of regression to the mean on the development and use of conditional reference values in children may be examined for analytes believed to be predictors of diseases in later life, as discussed in Section 5.4.1. The usefulness of subject-specific predictive methods, such as those mentioned in Section 7.3, may also be explored more generally. However, severe practical problems arise.

Foremost among these is the problem of transferrability of laboratory results. Current laboratory reporting systems have been primarily dedicated to serving a single institution. Whenever a patient is referred by a primary care physician to a regional hospital, it is common practice to have laboratory tests repeated in the laboratory of the hospital. Although such repeti-

1 MSH|^~\&|LAB|||199411122000702||ORU^R01||P|2.1|||<13>

2 PID||||123456^^^^B||NAME^PATIENT|||19351004|M|||||||||||987654321|||<13>

3 PV1|||MICU||<13>

4 ORC|RE|||||||||||||<13>

5 OBR||02908^000|402908-0-1|ABGR|||||||199411122000500||||||199411122000600|^2699||||T53704||||CHEM|||^^^^R|||||||||<13>

6 OBX|1|NM|PH^PH|1|7.38||(7.35-7.45)||||Z||<13>

7 OBX|2|NM|PCO2^PCO2|2|82|mm Hg|(35-45)|H^Y|||Z||<13>

8 OBX|3|NM|PO2^PO2|3|52|mm Hg|(75-100)|L^|||Z||<13>

9 OBX|4|NM|HCO3^BICARBONATE|4|48|mmol/L|(21-29)|H^|||Z||<13>

10 OBX|5|NM|BE^BASE EXCESS|5|19|mmol/L||||Z||<13>

11 OBX|6|ST|FIO2^FIO2|6|=85%|||||Z||<13>

Fig. 10.1 The laboratory results of a blood gas analysis as communicated by a laboratory information system to a hospital information system following the Health Level Seven (HL7) interface protocol. A sequence of 11 records is sent. Record 1 (MSH) is the message header record that carries information on the field separator character (|), encoding characters (^ ~\&), sending computer (LAB), date of the transaction (YYYYMMDDHHHHSS, November 22, 1994 at 0007:02 hours), the record type of the following records (ORU—observation results, unsolicited message; R01—segmented results), processing ID (P—production), and version ID (2.1). Each record is terminated with a carriage return character ⟨13⟩. Record 2 (PID), the patient identification record, carries information regarding the patient's ID number (123456), name (NAME ∧PATIENT), date of birth (YYYMMDD October 4, 1935), sex (M), and account code (987654321). Record 3 (PV1) is the patient visit record that gives the patient location (MICU). Record (ORC), the common order record, contains the order control code RE for results. Record 5 (OBR) is the observation request record, containing order numbers from the hospital information system (02908 ∧000 and 402908-0-1), the test identifier (ABGR), collection date and time (November 22, 1994 at 0005:00 hours), date and time specimen was received by laboratory (November 22, 1994 at 0006:00 hours, 1 minute later), the ordering physician code (2699), laboratory accession number (T53704), and the laboratory department performing the test (CHEM). Records 6 through 11 (OBX) contain results for the individual tests performed, pH, pCO2, pO2, bicarbonate, base excess, and FiO2. Each record has fields giving the result sequence number (1–6), result type (NM—numeric, ST—string), test code and full test name (e.g., HCO3 ∧BICARBONATE), subsequence number (1–6), the test result, the test reporting units (e.g., mm Hg), the test reference range, result flags (H—above upper reference limit, L—below lower reference limit), and observation result status (Z—complete). Note that the full HL7 standard (HL7 Technical Committee, 1994) contains many additional fields that are not used in the current example. These fields are expressed as "empty" fields (i.e., | |, two field separator characters with no intervening characters) in the example.

tion is not economical, it is dictated by wide variation among laboratories in analytical methods and reference values for the same tests. Laboratory scientists generally recognize this problem, but its solution has proved troublesome. Work is continuing to develop accurate methods and reference materials for laboratory testing, but until the standards emerging from these studies are widely adopted and generally implemented in clinical laboratories, there will still be variation among laboratories.

Fifteen years ago, Tietz (1979) described a model for a comprehensive measurement system in clinical chemistry. The hierarchical structure of this reference system consists of definitive reference and field (working) methods as well as appropriate reference materials. The function of the system is to transfer accuracy downward from the definitive method through the reference method to the field method and to provide traceability (assurance of transfer of accuracy and precision) from one component of the measurement system to another. Although the Tietz system has been widely accepted, there are still relatively few analytes for which definitive measurement methods have been described. Even in cholesterol, for which a definitive measurement method (isotope dilution mass spectroscopy) has been described, comparability of cholesterol measurements among laboratories remained relatively poor until the introduction of the National Cholesterol Education Program (NCEP) in 1988 and the stated goals of the NCEP Laboratory Standardization Panel (1990) to reduce cholesterol assay bias and imprecision to less than 3 percent within 5 years (see Chapter 8). Compliance with these goals by a majority of laboratories has been a gratifying demonstration that interlaboratory comparability can be achieved.

In tests for which a definitive method has not yet been described, standardization of laboratory results can be achieved by use of common standard reference materials. The Nordic protein project (Petersen et al., 1993) is an excellent example of how the use of a Certified Reference Material allowed the development and use of common reference intervals for nine specific plasma protein assays.

Another fundamental problem affecting the comparability of measurements over a long time period in a single patient involves the transient or long-term effects of drug therapy. Laboratory physicians have long been concerned with drug effects on laboratory test results (Young, 1990). Nonetheless, present computerized medical information systems do little to integrate information on the drugs a patient is taking with effects on test results. As more and more of the patient record becomes computerized and part of large, multi-patient data bases, there will be increasing opportunities to quantitate such effects more precisely. This may permit the compilation of tables of reference values adjusted for the effects of specific drugs.

10.3 INCREASING USE OF AUTOMATION

Steadily advancing capabilities in telecommunications, computing, and engineering have already had a profound effect on health care. For example, modern telecommunications technology enables medical information and images to be transmitted from a remote location (a rural area, for instance) to a center that provides specialty care. Such technology allows the specialist to interactively conduct and control the examination carried out at the remote site. In laboratory medicine, new generations of intelligent random-access laboratory instrumentation have streamlined clinical laboratory operations by providing "walk-away" capability (i.e., intelligence and self-diagnostic capacities built into the instrument that allow it to operate unattended for periods of time). Such capability frees the technologist to perform other functions during these times.

The introduction of robotic automation and advanced telecommunication techniques into the clinical laboratory points to the development of the integrated, fully automated laboratory as well as remote testing facilities placed at the actual site of medical care (point-of-care testing) but monitored at a central laboratory location by trained medical technologists. Laboratories in the 1990s are faced with the dilemma of providing quality services in the face of an expanding variety and number of analytical tests and reduced reimbursement rates. In an attempt to reduce labor costs, several leading laboratories have implemented new approaches to laboratory automation that employ robotic technology. These early efforts have been reviewed by Felder (1990, 1991).

Two major approaches to laboratory-wide automation have evolved from these pioneering uses of robots in clinical laboratories. One viewpoint holds that the use of standard industrial automation technology in the central laboratory is the best approach to improving efficiency and lowering labor costs. The best example of assembly-line laboratory automation can be found at the Kochi Medical School in Kochi, Japan (Sasaki, 1990, 1991) where an integrated automated system has been created beginning with phlebotomy and ending with tube disposal that operates with a minimum number of technologists. For example, Sasaki's clinical laboratory services a 600-bed hospital but requires only 25 technologists. A similar-sized laboratory in the United States requires five to eight times that number of employees.

The other viewpoint suggests that point-of-care testing will ultimately become the most cost-efficient way of providing laboratory tests. Data suggest that both these approaches can reduce laboratory costs while improving services. However, the point-of-care solution results in significant cost savings over a wide variety of settings where laboratory services are required: inpatient (bedside), outpatient clinic, physician's office, or even the shopping mall laboratory.

Workers at the University of Virginia have designed, built, and implemented a robotic workstation for the performance of point-of-care whole blood analysis in an unmanned critical care laboratory (Felder, 1991; Boyd et al., 1987, 1990). As an alternative to a complex centralized robotic processing area, these workers developed remote automated laboratory (RAL) systems for automating point-of-care testing in hospital intensive care units. The RAL is a laboratory analog of telemedicine systems in other disciplines.

The results from the analytical instruments at the satellite locations are sent to a central computer monitoring station via a network interface where results are viewed and either accepted or rejected by a trained medical technologist. The central monitoring station (satellite central) is located in the main clinical laboratory several floors away. Analysis of a specimen can be repeated, or the specimen can be discarded by the robot upon command from the central station. Technologists at satellite central can also shut down the satellite laboratory at any time in case of instrument failure.

Unmanned satellite laboratories represent a possible alternative to analysis in a central facility. They have been found to be cost-effective and have greatly reduced turnaround times for whole blood testing. Future development of these devices is foreseen for installation in outpatient clinics or small local hospital facilities and ultimately in physicians' offices.

10.3.1 Effects on Reference Values

Applications of telemedicine that make the specialist in a regional medical center available to the general practitioner, nurse practitioner, or physician's assistant at a distant site and point-of-care clinical laboratory facilities are both likely to have the same effect on the definition and use of reference values. This will be that conventional reference values based on healthy subject populations will gradually be replaced by context-sensitive reference points, that is, by values specifically intended to guide the physician in making the best decision with respect to the particular clinical condition he or she is involved in at the time. Such reference decision points would be included in computer-based expert systems or other optimizing algorithms for diagnosing and treating specific illnesses.

Many such systems have been developed during the past several decades; however, they have not yet found their way into general medical practice. Given more widespread application of telemedicine and the urgent desire for reduction of medical care costs, this situation may soon change. The vehicles for introducing the use of rule-based diagnosis and treatment algorithms, including associated reference points, will probably be what are now called "medical practice guidelines" (Bouhaddou et al. 1993; Sox, 1994).

The Omnibus Budget Reconciliation Act, passed by the U.S. Congress in 1989, mandated the creation of a system of decision rules called practice parameters to insure that appropriate and cost-effective medical actions were taken in various clinical circumstances. There is the expectation that promotion of medical practice guidelines will lead to the identification and reduction of unnecessary or inappropriate medical care. The anticipated enforcement of practice guidelines by linking physician compliance with the guidelines to payment has been a source of concern to clinicians who worry that guidelines will foster "cookbook medicine," decrease the autonomy and income of clinicians, and increase medico-legal liability. There are additional concerns that rigid enforcement of guidelines may harm patients, interfere with individualized care, increase costs, and promote unfair judgments against those who deviate from the guidelines for good reasons. Because guidelines are bound to be imperfect, Woolf (1993) proposed a model that links the intensity of enforcement to the scientific and clinical quality of each guideline.

10.3.2 Example

As an example of how practice guidelines may change present concepts of reference values, we consider the diagnosis and management of asymptomatic primary hyperparathyroidism. This subject was recently considered at a consensus development conference sponsored by the National Institutes of Health, and a consensus statement was issued (Consensus Development Conference Panel, 1991). The full proceedings of the conference were published soon afterwards.

Although the diagnosis of primary hyperparathyroidism is established by persistent hypercalcemia with an elevated serum parathyroid hormone concentration, and parathyroidectomy cures the disease, recent studies have shown that hyperparathyroidism can be managed conservatively in many cases. Conservative management is based on the following line of reasoning. First, there is evidence that prolonged elevated concentrations of parathyroid hormone do not necessarily lead to clinically significant osteoporosis, a disease characterized by large reduction in bone mineral mass with associated bone fragility. Second, studies in which patients have been followed on conservative management have shown little evidence of disease progression or deterioration of renal function. Third, many patients with hyperparathyroidism are elderly, have cardiovascular disease, and are poor candidates for surgery.

Because parathyroid surgery may not produce better results than conservative management in many patients and entails both risk and expense, the consensus panel recommended conservative management in patients with a calcium concentration that is only mildly elevated (0.25–0.40 mmol/L, or 1.0–1.6 mg/dL) above the upper reference limit with no prior episodes of life-threatening hypercalcemia and normal renal and bone status. Conversely, surgery is recommended in patients with markedly elevated serum calcium concentrations (>3 mmol/L, or 12 mg/dL), a prior episode of life-threatening hypercalcemia, a reduced creatinine clearance (30 percent below those of age-matched reference subjects with normal renal function), a markedly elevated 24-hour urinary calcium excretion (>400 mg/24 hr), or a substantially reduced bone mass (>2 standard deviations below those of age-gender-race- matched controls).

A serum calcium concentration above 2.6 mmol/L (10.4 mg/ dL) is considered abnormal by most physicians, but the practice guideline described above sets a new threshold of 3.0 mmol/L (12 mg/dL) before possible initiation of surgical management. This new threshold is based on studies of the outcomes of patients with hyperparathyroidism who were managed conservatively.[1] Such research on the outcomes of various clinical treat-

---

[1] We are talking here about appropriate levels of serum calcium for deciding between different courses of management of patients with

ments is becoming more prevalent and will be utilized in the elaboration of future practice guidelines. As in serum cholesterol, the resulting decision thresholds will be based on analysis of outcomes research data rather than on the traditional 97.5th percentile of the distribution of reference values in healthy subjects. To what extent medical costs will enter the analysis of such data is not currently known, but it not hard to conceive of the derivation of "economically efficient" reference values that optimize the cost-effectiveness of practice guidelines.

10.4 ADVANCES IN MOLECULAR GENETICS

The introduction of new techniques in molecular genetics over the past 10 years has revolutionized medical knowledge of disease. As these techniques are refined and more of the human genome is understood, an increasing number of genetic conditions may be shown to have an influence on laboratory results. Eventually, it may be necessary to define gene-adjusted as well as age- and gender-adjusted reference values.

As an example, consider the genetic variant of apolipoprotein A1 known as Apo A1$_{Milano}$.[2] Apo A1$_{Milano}$ was originally

---

diagnosed hyperparathyroidism. In Chapter 8, we referred to the work of Groth et al. (1983) on optimal reference values for serum calcium in discriminating between the diagnoses of hyperparathyroidism and hypercalcemia due to malignancy.

[2] Apolipoproteins are the protein components of lipoprotein particles that carry lipids in the blood. They comprise a heterogeneous group of about 13 major human plasma apolipoproteins. Apolipoproteins have several characteristics that make them interesting potential markers of lipid disorders. First, apolipoproteins represent the only genetically determined components of lipoproteins. They play an important structural role in the biosynthesis/secretion of lipoproteins. They are responsible for the activation of enzymes known to be important in lipid metabolism, and they are instrumental in the interaction of lipoproteins with cellular receptors. In clinical studies of adults, coronary artery disease has been shown to be positively associated

described in an extensive Italian kindred from the village of Limone su Garda. Members of this kindred were found to have HDL cholesterol concentrations approximately 33 percent of normal associated with an electrophoretic variant of Apo A1 that was named Apo A1$_{Milano}$. In spite of low HDL cholesterol levels, individuals in this kindred have no symptomatology. In particular, they show no increased incidence of atherosclerotic disease when compared with close relatives without the Apo A1 variant. Thus, Apo A1$_{Milano}$ represents a genetic variant that affects serum HDL cholesterol concentrations but has no apparent other effects. Although Apo A1$_{Milano}$ represents a fascinating entity for lipid researchers, it is of little clinical consequence except for creating confusion in interpreting the associated low HDL cholesterol concentrations. If it were known that an individual carried the Apo A1$_{Milano}$ variant, it would be reasonable to adjust the reference values used to interpret HDL cholesterol concentrations in this individual. There will likely be many other genetically determined traits that have an influence on laboratory analytes. As these become recognized, the more specific information they provide may allow us to define more informative reference values.

10.5 FINAL REMARKS

Modern currents of change in the practice of laboratory medicine are probably indicators of change in medical practice as a whole. They come sooner in laboratory medicine because clinical laboratorians have much longer and deeper experience than other medical professionals with the interpretation of quantitative data, the development of computerized information systems, and the promises and problems of information transfer. Probably more than others in the health care field, they are

---

with apolipoprotein B, the principal protein of low-density lipoprotein (LDL) particles, and inversely correlated with apolipoprotein A1, the principal protein of high-density lipoprotein (HDL) particles.

vulnerable to the demands of cost reduction and more capable of responding to these pressures in innovative ways.

With respect to reference values in the practice of laboratory medicine and medical care in general, we have called attention specifically to two forces that will undoubtedly grow stronger in coming years. One of these is outcomes research leading to the establishment (probably by consensus of experts) of cutpoints of risk for a given analyte predictive of a given disease or category of closely related diseases. Each of these cutpoints will be associated with a recommended course of medical action. As we have seen in the case of serum cholesterol, such cutpoints may have little correlation with conventional reference limits but will necessarily make more stringent demands on analytical accuracy.

The other force is the integrated medical record that will emphasize the need for objective, sequential study of serial measurements. Again, conventional reference limits will be replaced, this time by patient-specific predictive models and values. The effects of genetic mechanisms and environmental influences will be automatically reflected in individual serial records. As we mentioned, the problem of tranferrability will loom especially large here, again putting very stringent demands on analytical accuracy (especially the absence of bias) regardless of which measurement devices are used.

Finally, we will undoubtedly see a continuing addition of new analytes to be measured. Advances in the molecular biology of disease have already added new specific proteins to the list that require new and more precise measurement techniques. The kinds of measurements made and the units of measurement may change, but we expect that the same statistical problems will remain. We hope that this book has provided some useful tools to help in defining these problems clearly and to move toward their resolution.

REFERENCES

Abramowitz, M., and Stegun, I. A., eds. (1964). *Handbook of Mathematical Functions.* U.S. Department of Commerce, National Bureau of Standards, Washington, D.C., p. 932 (26.2.16).

Accuracy and Precision Goals in Clinical Chemistry Testing: Can They Be Defined by Medical Relevance? (1993). (Clinical Chemistry Forum, R. Rej, ed.) *Clin. Chem. 39,* 1446–1544.

Albert, A. (1981). Atypicality indices as reference values for laboratory data. *Amer. J. Clin. Pathol. 76,* 421–425.

Albert, A. (1982). On the use and computation of likelihood ratios in clinical chemistry. *Clin. Chem. 28,* 1113–1119.

Albert, A., and Harris, E. K. (1987). *Multivariate Interpretation of Clinical Laboratory Data.* Marcel Dekker, New York.

Alström, T. (1981). Evolution and nomenclature of the reference value concept. In *Reference Values in Laboratory Medicine,* R. Gräsbeck and T. Alström, eds. Wiley, New York, pp. 3–13.

Altman, D. G. (1993). Construction of age-related reference centiles using absolute residuals. *Statist. Med. 12,* 917–924.

325

Amador, E., and Hsi, B. P. (1969). Indirect methods for estimating the normal range. *Amer. J. Clin. Pathol. 52*, 538–546.

Barnett, G. O., Jenders R. A., and Chueh H. C. (1993). The computer-based clinical record—where do we stand? *Ann. Intern. Med. 119*, 1046–1048.

Barnett, R. N. (1989). Error limits and quality control (editorial). *Arch. Pathol. Lab. Med. 115*, 829–830.

Barnett, V., and Lewis T. (1994). *Outliers in Statistical Data*, 3rd. ed. Wiley, New York.

Barrett, A. E., Cameron, S. J., Fraser, C. G., et al. (1979). A clinical view of analytical goals in clinical biochemistry. *J. Clin. Pathol. 32*, 893–896.

Bartlett, M. S. (1947). The use of transformations. *Biometrics 3*, 39–52.

Becktel, J. M. (1970). Simplified estimation of normal ranges from routine laboratory data. *Clin. Chim. Acta 28*, 119–125.

Belk, W. P., and Sunderman, F. W. (1947). A survey of the accuracy of chemical analyses in clinical laboratories. *Amer. J. Clin. Pathol. 17*, 853–861.

Benson, E. S. (1972). The concept of the normal range. *Hum. Pathol. 3*, 152–155.

Berg, B., Nilsson, J. E., Solberg, H. E., and Tryding, N. (1981). Practical experience in the selection and preparation of reference individuals: empirical testing of the provisional Scandinavian recommendations. In *Reference Values in Laboratory Medicine*, R. Gräsbeck and T. Alström, Eds. Wiley, New York, pp. 55–64.

Bhattacharya, C. (1967). A simple method of resolution of a distribution into Gaussian components. *Biometrics 23*, 115– 135.

Bokelund, H., Winkel, P., and Statland, B. E. (1974). Factors contributing to intra-individual variation of serum constituents. 3. Use of randomized duplicate serum specimens to evaluate sources of analytical error. *Clin. Chem. 20*, 1507–1512.

Bouhaddou, O., Frucci, L., Cofrin, K., Larsen, D., Warner, H., Jr, Huber, P., Sorenson, D., Turner, C., and Warner H. (1993). Implementation of practice guidelines in a clinical setting using a computerized knowledge base (Iliad). *Proc. Annu. Symp. Comput. Appl. Med. Care*, 258–262.

Box, G. E. P., and Cox, D. R. (1964). An analysis of transformations. *J. Roy. Statist. Soc. B26*, 211–252.

Box, G. E. P. and Jenkins, G. M. (1970). *Time Series Analysis*. Holden-Day, San Francisco.

Boyd, J. C., and Lacher, D. A. (1982a). The multivariate reference range: an alternative interpretation of multi-test profiles. *Clin. Chem. 28*, 259–265.

Boyd, J. C., and Lacher, D. A. (1982b). A multi-stage Gaussian transformation algorithm for clinical laboratory data. *Clin. Chem. 28*, 1735–1741.

Boyd, J. C., and Harris, E. K. (1986). Utility of reference changes for the monitoring of inpatient laboratory data. In *Optimal Use of the Clinical Laboratory*, O. Zinder, ed. Karger, Basel.

Boyd J. C., Felder R. A., Margrey K. S., Martinez A., and Savory J. (1987). Use of a robotic arm for specimen handling in a remote, unmanned clinical chemistry laboratory. *Clin. Chem. 33*, 1560–1561.

Boyd J. C., Felder R. A., Margrey K. S., Martinez A., Vaughn D., and Savory J. (1990) Critical care testing using unmanned robotic facilities. In *Automation and New Technology in the Clinical Laboratory*, K. Okuda ed., Blackwell Scientific, Oxford, pp. 93–96.

Brown, R. G. (1962). *Smoothing, Forecasting, and Prediction of Discrete Time Series*. Prentice-Hall, Englewood Cliffs, NJ.

Burnett, R. W. (1975). Accurate estimation of standard deviations for quantitative methods used in clinical chemistry. *Clin. Chem. 21*, 1935–1938.

Burton, M. E., Vasko, M. R., and Brater, D. C. (1985). Comparison of drug dosing methods. *Clin. Pharmacokinet. 10*, 1–37.

Cameron, N. (1980). Conditional standards for growth in height of British children from 5.0 to 15.99 years of age. *Ann. Hum. Biol. 7*, 331–337.

Campbell, B. G. (1989). Evaluation of two types of "medically significant error limits" and two quality control procedures on a multi-channel analyzer. *Arch. Pathol. Lab. Med. 113*, 834–837.

Campbell, D. G., and Owen, J. A. (1967). Clinical laboratory error in perspective. *Clin. Biochem. 1*, 3–11.

Caudill, S. P., and Boone, D.J. (1986). Analytical variance and definition of a reference change as a function of calcium concentration. *Clin. Chem. 32*, 308–313.

Chambers, J. M., Cleveland, W. S., Kleiner, B., and Tukey, P. A. (1983). *Graphical Methods for Data Analysis*. Duxbury Press, Boston.

Chew, V. (1966). Confidence, prediction, and tolerance regions for the multivariate normal distribution. *J. Amer. Statist. Assoc. 61*, 605–617.

Chiou, W. L., Gadalla, M. A. F., and Peng, G. W. (1978). Method for rapid estimation of the total body drug clearance and adjustment of dosage regimens in patients during a constant-rate intravenous infusion. *J. Pharmacokinet. Biopharmaceut. 6*, 135–151.

Cleveland, W. S. (1979). Robust locally weighted regression and smoothing scatterplots. *J. Amer. Statist. Assoc. 74*, 829–836.

Cochran, W. S. (1941). The distribution of the largest of a set of estimated variances as a fraction of their total. *Ann. Eugen. 11*, 47–52.

Cole, T. J. (1988). Fitting smoothed centile curves to reference data (with discussion). *J. Roy. Statist. Soc. A151*, 385–418.

Cole, T. J., and Green, P.J. (1992). Smoothing reference centile curves: the LMS method and penalized likelihood. *Statist. Med. 11*, 1305–1319.

College of American Pathologists. (CAP) (1977). *Analytical Goals in Clinical Chemistry*. Proceedings of the 1976 Aspen Conference on Analytical Goals in Clinical Chemistry, F. R. Elevitch, ed.

College of American Pathologists (1988). *Evaluation of Proficiency Testing Results for Quantitative Methods in Relation to Clinical Usefulness*. Conference XIII. *Arch. Pathol. Lab. Med. 112*, 327–474.

Consensus Development Conference Panel (1991). Diagnosis and management of asymptomatic primary hyperparathyroidism:

consensus development conference statement. *Ann. Intern. Med.* 114, 593–597.

Cooper, G. R., Myers, G. L., Smith, S. J., and Schlant, R. C. (1992). Blood lipid measurements: variations and practical utility. *J. Amer. Med. Assoc.* 267, 1652–1660.

Cooper, G. R., Smith, S. J., Myers, G. L., et al. (1994). Estimating and minimizing effects of biologic sources of variation by relative range when measuring the mean of serum lipids and lipoproteins. *Clin. Chem.* 40, 227–232.

Costongs, G. M. P. T., Janson, P. C. W., Hermans, J., et al. (1985). Short-term and long-term intra-individual variations and critical differences of clinical chemical laboratory parameters. *J. Clin. Chem. Clin. Biochem.* 23, 7–16.

Cotlove, E., Harris, E. K., and Williams, G. Z. (1970). Biological and analytic components of variation in long-term studies of serum consituents in normal subjects. III. Physiological and medical implications. *Clin. Chem.* 16, 1028–1032.

Cox, D. R. (1961). Prediction by exponentially weighted moving averages and related methods. *J. Roy. Statist. Soc.*, B23, 414-422.

Cummings, S. T., and Fraser, C.G. (1989). Total amylase and pancreatic isoamylase in serum and urine: considerations from data on biological variation. *Ann. Clin. Biochem.* 26, 335–340.

D'Argenio, D. Z., and Khakmahd, K. (1983). Adaptive control of theophylline therapy: importance of blood sampling times. *J. Pharmacokinet. and Biopharmaceut.* 11, 547–559.

Davis, C. E. (1976). The effect of regression to the mean in epidemiologic and clinical studies. *Amer. J. Epidemiol.* 104, 493–498.

Deming, W. E. (1950). *Some Theory of Sampling.* Wiley, New York.

Dick, R. S., and Steen, E. B. (1991). *The Computer-Based Patient Record: An Essential Technology for Health Care.* National Academy Press, Washington, D.C.

Dixon, W. J. (1953). Processing data for outliers. *Biometrics 9*, 74–89.

Dixon, W. J., and Massey, F. J., Jr. (1983). *Introduction to Statistical Analysis*, 4th ed. McGraw-Hill, New York.

Documenta Geigy Scientific Tables, 7th ed. (1970). J. R. Geigy, Basel.

Doodson, A. T. (1917). Relation of mode, median and mean in frequency curves. Biometrika 11, 425–429.

Durbridge, T. C. (1983). Clinical acceptance of a multi-test reference region for biochemical-panel results. Clin. Chem. 29, 1724–1726.

Efron, B. (1979). Bootstrap methods: another look at the jackknife. Ann. Statist. 7, 1–26.

Efron B. (1982). The Jackknife, the Bootstrap and Other Resampling Plans. Society for Industrial and Applied Mathematics, Philadelphia.

Elion-Gerritzen, W. E. (1980). Analytic precision in clinical chemistry and medical decisions. Amer. J. Clin. Pathol. 73, 183–195.

Elveback, L. R. (1972). How high is high? A proposed alternative to the normal range. Mayo Clin. Proc. 47, 93–97.

Elveback, L. R., and Taylor, W.F. (1969). Statistical methods of estimating percentiles. Ann. N.Y. Acad. Sci. 161, 538–548.

Elveback, L. R., Guiller, C. L., and Keating, F. R. Jr. (1970). Health, normality, and the ghost of Gauss. J. Amer. Med. Assoc. 211, 69–75.

Essin D. J. (1993). Intelligent processing of loosely structured documents as a strategy for organizing electronic health care records. Meth. Inform. Med. 32, 265–268.

Faulkner, W. R., and Meites, S., eds. (1994). Geriatric Clinical Chemistry: Reference Values. AACC Press, Washington, D.C.

Felder R. A., Boyd J. C., Margrey K., Holman W., and Savory J. (1990). Robotics in the medical laboratory. Clin. Chem. 36, 1–10.

Felder R. A., Boyd J. C., Margrey K. S., Holman W., Roberts J., and Savory J. (1991). Robots in health care. Anal. Chem. 63, 741A–747A.

Flynn, F. V., Piper, K. A. J., Garcia-Webb, P., et al. (1974). The frequency distributions of commonly determined blood constituents in healthy blood donors. Clin. Chim. Acta 52, 163–171.

Flynn, F. V., Piper, K. A. J., Garcia-Webb, P., et al. (1976). Biological and analytical variation of commonly determined blood constituents in healthy blood donors. Clin. Chim. Acta 70, 179–189.

Ford, R. P., Mitchell, P. E. G., and Fraser, C. G. (1988). Desirable performance characteristics and clinical utility of immunoglobulin and light-chain assays derived from data on biological variation. *Clin. Chem. 34,* 1733–1736.

Fraser, C.G. (1981). Analytical goals in clinical biochemistry. In *Progress in Clinical Pathology, Vol. 8,* M. Stefanini and E. S. Benson, eds. Grune & Stratton, New York, pp. 101–122.

Fraser, C. G. (1983). Desirable performance standards for clinical chemistry tests. *Adv. Clin. Chem. 23,* 299–339.

Fraser, C. G. (1987). Desirable standards of performance for therapeutic drug monitoring. *Clin. Chem. 33,* 387–389.

Fraser, C. G. (1988). The application of theoretical goals based on biological variation data in proficiency testing. *Arch. Pathol. Lab. Med. 112,* 404–415.

Fraser, C. G., and Harris, E. K. (1989). Generation and application of data on biological variation in clinical chemistry. *CRC Crit. Rev. Clin. Lab. Sci. 27,* 409–437.

Fraser, C. G., and Lipworth, B. J. (1988). More on analytical goals for theophylline assays. *Clin. Chem. 34,* 796–797.

Fraser, C. G., and Petersen, P. H. (1993). Desirable standards for laboratory tests if they are to fulfill medical needs. *Clin. Chem. 39,* 1447–1455.

Fraser, C. G., Petersen, P. H., and Larsen, M. L. (1990). Setting analytical goals for random analytical error in specific clinical monitoring situations. *Clin. Chem. 36,* 1625–1628.

Frisse M. E., Schnase J. L., and Metcalfe E. S. (1994). Models for patient records. *Acad. Med. 69,* 546–550.

Fulwood, R., Rifkind, B. M., Havlik, R. J., et al. (1987). Trends in serum cholestrol levels among US adults aged 20 to 74 years. *J. Amer. Med. Assoc. 257,* 937–942.

Galen, R. S., and Gambino, S. R. (1975). *Beyond Normality: The Predictive Value and Efficiency of Medical Diagnoses.* Wiley, New York.

Gillard, B. K., Simbala, J. A., and Goodglick, L. (1983). Reference intervals for amylase isoenzymes in serum and plasma of infants and children. *Clin. Chem. 29,* 1119–1123.

Gindler, E. M. (1970). Calculation of normal ranges by methods used for resolution of overlapping Gaussian distributions. *Clin. Chem* 16, 124–128.

Gnanadesikan, R., and Kettenring, J. R. (1972). Robust estimates, residuals and outlier detection with multiresponse data. *Biometrics* 28, 81–124.

Gottmann, A. W., Nosanchuk, J. S., and Anderson, G. S. (1976). Long-term quality-control charting: a simple method. *Clin. Chem.* 22, 270–272.

Gowans, E. M. S., and Fraser, C. G. (1988). Biological variation of serum and urine creatinine and creatinine clearance: ramifications for interpretation of results and patient care. *Ann. Clin. Biochem.* 25, 259–263.

Gowans, E. M. S., Petersen, P. H., Blaabjerg, O., and Hørder, M. (1988). Analytical goals for the acceptance of common reference intervals for laboratories throughout a geographical area. *Scand. J. Clin. Lab. Invest.* 48, 757–764.

Grams, R. R., Johnson, E. A., and Benson, E. S. (1972). Laboratory data analysis system: Section III—multivariate normality. *Amer. J. Clin. Pathol.* 58, 188–200.

Gräsbeck, R. (1978). Terminology and biological aspects of reference values. In *Logic and Economics of Clinical Laboratory Use*, E. Benson and M. Rubin, eds. Elsevier, New York, pp. 77–90.

Gräsbeck, R., and Saris, N.-E. (1969). Establishment and use of normal values. *Scand. J. Clin. Lab. Invest.* 24 (Suppl. 110), 62–63.

Griffiths, D. A. (1980). Interval estimation of the three-parameter lognormal distribution via the likelihood function. *Appl. Statist.* 29, 58–68.

Groth, T. (1984). The role of formal biodynamic models in laboratory medicine. *Scand. J. Clin. Lab. Invest.* 44 (Suppl. 171), 175–192.

Groth, T., and de Verdier, C.-H. (1982). Biodynamic models as preprocessors of clinical laboratory data. In *Advanced Interpretation of Clinical Laboratory Data*, C. Heusghem, A. Albert, and E. Benson, eds., Marcel Dekker, New York, pp. 151–170.

Groth, T., Ljunghall, S., and de Verdier, C.-H. (1983). Optimal screening for patients with hyperparathyroidism with use of serum calcium observations. A decision-theoretical analysis. *Scand. J. Clin. Lab. Invest. 43*, 699–707.

Gullick. H. D., and Schauble, M. K. (1972). SD unit system for standardized reporting and interpretation of laboratory data. *Amer. J. Clin. Pathol. 57*, 517–525.

Gumbel, E. J. (1961). Bivariate logistic distributions. *J. Amer. Statist. Assoc. 56*, 335–349.

Hadi, A. S. (1992). Identifying multiple outliers in multivariate data. *J. Roy. Statist. Soc. B54*, 761–771.

Halkin, H., Mazar, S., Almog, S., and Schnaps, Y. (1982). Components of variability in serum theophylline concentrations during maintenance therapy with a sustained release formulation. *Br. J. Clin. Pharmacol. 23*, 225–228.

Hallworth, M. J. (1988). Audit of therapeutic drug monitoring. *Ann. Clin. Biochem. 25*, 121–128.

Harrell, F. E., and Davis, C.E. (1982). A new distribution-free quantile estimator. *Biometrika 69*, 635–640.

Harris, E. K. (1970). Distinguishing physiologic variation from analytic variation. *J. Chron. Dis. 23*, 469–480.

Harris, E. K. (1974). Effects of intra- and interindividual variation on the appropriate use of normal ranges. *Clin. Chem. 20*, 1535–1542.

Harris, E. K. (1979). Statistical principles underlying analytical goal-setting in clinical chemistry. *Amer. J. Clin. Pathol. 72*, 374–382.

Harris, E. K. (1981). Statistical aspects of reference values in clinical pathology. In *Progress in Clinical Pathology*, Vol. 8, Mario Stefanini and Ellis S. Benson, eds. Grune & Stratton, New York, pp. 45–66.

Harris, E. K. (1988). Proposed goals for analytic precision and accuracy in single-point diagnostic testing: theoretical basis and comparison with data from College of American Pathologists Proficiency Surveys. *Arch. Pathol. Lab. Med. 112*, 416–420.

Harris, E. K., and Boyd, J. C. (1990). On dividing reference data into subgroups to produce separate reference ranges. *Clin. Chem. 36*, 265–270.

Harris, E. K., and Brown, S. S. (1979). Temporal changes in the concentrations of serum constituents in healthy men. *Ann. Clin. Biochem. 16*, 169–176.

Harris, E. K., and DeMets, D. L. (1972a). Effects of intra- and interindividual variation on distributions of single measurements. *Clin. Chem. 18*, 244–249.

Harris, E. K., and DeMets, D. L. (1972b). Estimation of normal ranges and cumulative proportions by transforming observed distributions to Gaussian form. *Clin. Chem. 18*, 605–612.

Harris, E. K., and Yasaka, T. (1983). On the calculation of a "reference change" for comparing two consecutive measurements. *Clin. Chem. 29*, 25–30.

Harris, E. K., Kanofsky, P., Shakarji, G., and Cotlove E. (1970). Biological and analytic components of variation in long-term studies of serum constituents in normal subjects. II. Estimating biological components of variation. *Clin. Chem. 16*, 1022–1027.

Harris, E. K., Cooil, B. K., Shakarji, G., and Williams, G. Z. (1980). On the use of statistical models of within-person variation in long-term studies of healthy individuals. *Clin. Chem. 26*, 383–391.

Harris, E. K., Yasaka T., Horton, M. R., and Shakarji, G. (1982). Comparing multivariate and univariate subject-specific reference regions for blood constituents in healthy persons. *Clin. Chem. 28*, 422–426.

Harris, E. K., Wong, E. T., and Shaw, S. T. (1991). Statistical criteria for separate reference intervals: race and gender groups in creatine kinase. *Clin. Chem. 37*, 1580–1582.

Harrison, P. J., and Stevens, C. F. (1976). Bayesian forecasting (with discussion). *J. Roy. Statist. Soc. B38*, 205–247.

Hart, B. I. (1942). Significance levels for the ratio of the mean square successive difference to the variance. *Ann. Math. Stat. 13*, 445–447.

Harville, D. A. (1977). Maximum likelihood approaches to variance component estimation and related problems. *J. Amer. Stat. Assoc.* 72, 341–353.

Healy, M. J. R. (1962). The effect of age-grouping on the distribution of a measurement affected by growth. *Amer. J. Phys. Anthropol.* 20, 49–50.

Healy, M. J. R. (1968). Multivariate normal plotting. *Appl. Stat.* 17, 157–161.

Healy, M. J. R. (1969a). Rao's paradox concerning multivariate tests of significance. *Biometrics* 25, 411–413.

Healy, M. J. R. (1969b). Normal values from a statistical viewpoint. *Bull. Acad. Roy. Med. Belg.* 9, 703–718.

Healy, M. J. R. (1979a). Outliers in clinical chemistry quality-control schemes. *Clin. Chem.* 25, 675–677.

Healy, M. J. R. (1979b). Some statistical paradoxes of the normal range. In *Evaluation of Efficacy of Medical Action*, A. Alperovitch, F. T. de Dombal, F. Gremy, eds. North-Holland, Amsterdam, pp. 509–514.

Healy, M. J. R., Rasbash, J., and Yang, M. (1988). Distribution-free estimation of age-related centiles. *Ann. Hum. Biol.* 15, 17–22.

Hendeles, L., and Weinberger, M. (1981). Theophylline: therapeutic use and serum concentration monitoring. In *Individualizing Drug Therapy*, Vol 1, W. J. Taylor, and A. L. Finn, eds. Gross, Townsend, Frank, New York.

Henry, R. J. (1960). Improper statistics characterizing the normal range. *Amer. J. Clin. Pathol.* 34, 326–327.

Herrera, L. (1958). The precision of percentiles in establishing normal limits in medicine. *J. Lab. Clin. Med.* 52, 34–42.

Hill, P. D. (1985). Kernel estimation of a distribution function. *Commun. Statist. Theor. Meth.* 14, 605–620.

HL7 Technical Committee (1994). *Health Level Seven: An Application Protocol for Electronic Data Exchange in Health Care Environments.* Version 2.2. Ann Arbor, MI.

Hoffmann, R. G. (1963). Statistics in the practice of medicine. *J. Amer. Med. Assoc.* 185, 864–873.

Holt, C. C. (1957). *Forecasting Trends and Seasonals by Exponentially Weighted Moving Averages*. ONR Memorandum No. 52, Carnegie Institute of Technology, Pittsburgh.

Hölzel, W. G. E. (1987a). Intra-individual variation of some analytes in serum of patients with insulin-dependent diabetes mellitus. *Clin. Chem.* 33, 57–61.

Hölzel, W. G. E. (1987b). Intra-individual variation of some analytes in serum of patients with chronic renal failure. *Clin. Chem.* 33, 670–673.

Hölzel, W. G. E. (1987c). Intra-individual variation of some analytes in serum from patients with chronic liver diseases. *Clin. Chem.* 33, 1133–1136.

Hölzel, W. G. E. (1988). Influence of hypertension and antihypertensive drugs on the biological intra-individual variation of electrolytes and lipids in serum. *Clin. Chem.* 34, 1485–1488.

Homburger, H. A., and Hewan-Lowe, K. (1979). Predictive values of thyroxine, thyrotropin, and triiodothryonine concentrations in serum. *Clin. Chem.* 25, 669–674.

Howey, J. E. A., Browning, M. C. K., and Fraser, C.G. (1987). Selecting the optimum specimen for assessing slight albuminuria, and a strategy for clinical investigation: novel uses of data on biological variation. *Clin. Chem.* 33, 2034–2038.

Hyltoft-Petersen P., Blaabjerg O., Irjala K., Icen A., and Bjoro K. (1993). A model for quality achievement: the Nordic Protein project. *Scand. J. Clin. Lab. Invest.* 53 (Suppl. 212), 10–12.

International Federation of Clinical Chemistry (IFCC) Expert Panel on Theory of Reference Values: The Theory of Reference Values. Part 1. (1979): The concept of reference values. *J. Clin. Chem. Clin. Biochem.* 17 ,337–339; Part 2. (1984): Selection of individuals for the production of reference values. *J. Clin. Chem. Clin. Biochem.* 22, 203–208; Part 3. (1988): Preparation of individuals and collection of specimens for the production of reference values. *J. Clin. Chem. Clin. Biochem.* 26, 593–598; Part 5. (1987): Statistical treatment of collected reference values. Determination of reference limits. *J. Clin. Chem. Clin. Biochem.* 25, 645–656.

Irjala, K., Koskinen, P., Icen, A., and Palosuo, T. (1990). Reference intervals for immunoglobulins IgA, IgG and IgM in serum in adults and in children aged 6 months to 14 years. *Scand. J. Clin. Lab. Invest. 50*, 573–577.

Isaacs, D., Altman, D. G., Tidmarsh, C. E., et al. (1983). Serum immunoglobulin concentrations in preschool children measured by laser nephelometry: reference ranges for IgG, IgA, IgM. *J. Clin. Pathol. 36*, 1193–1196.

James, K. E. (1973). Regression toward the mean in uncontrolled clinical studies. *Biometrics 29*, 121–130.

Jenny, R. W. (1991). Analytical goals for determinations of theophylline concentration in serum. *Clin. Chem. 37*, 154–158.

John, J. A., and Draper, N. R. (1980). An alternate family of transformations. *Appl. Statist. 29*, 190–197.

Johnson, N. L. (1949). Systems of frequency curves generated by methods of translation. *Biometrika 36*, 149–176.

Johnson, N. L., and Kotz, S. (1972). Bivariate and trivariate normal distributions. In *Distributions in Statistics: Continuous Multivariate Distributions*. Wiley, New York, p. 88 (Chap. 36).

Johnson, R. A., and Wichern, D. W. (1988). *Applied Multivariate Statistical Analysis*, 2nd Ed. Prentice-Hall, Englewood Cliffs, NJ.

Jones, R. H. (1981). Fitting continuous-time autoregressions to discrete data. In *Applied Time Series Analysis*, II, D. F. Finley, ed. Academic Press, New York, pp. 651–682.

Jones, R. H. (1985). Time series analysis with unequally spaced data. In *Handbook of Statistics, Vol. 5: Time Series in the Time Domain*. E. J. Hannan, P. R. Krishnaiah, and M. M. Rao, eds. North-Holland, New York, pp. 157–177.

Jones, R. H., and Ackerson, L. M. (1990). Serial correlation in unequally spaced longitudinal data. *Biometrika 77*, 721–731.

Jones, R. H., and Boadi-Boateng, F. (1991). Unequally spaced longitudinal data with AR(1) serial correlation. *Biometrics 47*, 161–175.

Kägedal. B., Sandström, A., and Tibbling G. (1978). Determination of a trivariate reference region for free thyroxine index, free triiodothyronine index, and thyrotropin from results obtained in a health survey of middle-aged women. *Clin. Chem. 24*, 1744–1750.

Kägedal, B., Larsson, L., Norr, A., and Toss, G. (1982). Trivariate evaluation of a thyroid hormone panel in clinical practice compared with multiple univariate evaluation. *Scand. J. Clin. Lab. Invest.* 42, 177–180.

Kairisto, V., Virtanen, A., Uusipaikka, E., et al. (1993). Method for determining reference changes from patients' serial data: example of cardiac enzymes. *Clin. Chem.* 39, 2298–2304.

Keating, F. R. Jr., Jones, J. D., Elveback, L. R., and Randall, R. V. (1969). The relation of age and sex to distribution of values in healthy adults of serum calcium, inorganic phosphorus, magnesium alkaline phosphatase, total proteins, albumin and blood urea. *J. Lab. Clin. Med.* 73, 825–834.

Kelman, A. W., Whiting, B., and Bryson, S. M. (1982). OPT: a package of computer programs for parameter optimization in clinical pharmacokinetics. *Br. J. Clin. Pharmac.* 14, 247–256.

Keyser, J. W. (1965). The concept of the normal range in clinical chemistry. *Postgrad. Med. J.* 41, 443–447.

Klee, G. G. (1993). Tolerance limits for short-term analytical bias and analytical imprecision derived from clinical assay specificity. *Clin. Chem.* 39, 1514–1518.

Lacher, D. A., and Connelly, D. P. (1988). Rate and delta checks compared for selected chemistry tests. *Clin. Chem.* 34, 1966–1970.

Ladenson, J. H. (1975). Patients as their own controls: use of the computer to identify "laboratory error." *Clin. Chem.* 21, 1648–1653.

Laird, N. M., and Ware, J. H. (1982). Random-effects models for longitudinal data. *Biometrics 38*, 963–974.

Larsen, M. L., Blaabjerg, O., Petersen, P. H., et al. (1990). Analytical goal setting prior to selection of a method for glycated haemoglobin. *Scand. J. Clin. Lab. Invest. 50*, 715–721.

Larsen, M. L., Fraser, C. G., and Petersen, P. H. (1991). A comparison of analytical goals for haemoglobin A_{1c} assays derived using different strategies. *Ann. Clin. Biochem. 28*, 272–278.

Linnet, K. (1987). Two-stage transformation systems for normalization of reference distributions evaluated. *Clin. Chem. 33*, 381–386.

Linnet, K. (1988). Testing normality of transformed data. *Appl. Statist.* 37, 180–186.

Linnet, K. (1989). Choosing quality-control systems to detect maximum clinically allowable analytical errors. *Clin. Chem.* 35, 284–288.

Lucas, J. M. (1982). Combined Shewhart-CUSUM quality control schemes. *J. Qual. Technol.* 14, 51–59.

Mahalanobis, P. C. (1936). On the generalized distance in statistics. *Proc. Nat. Inst. Sci. (India)* 12, 49–55.

Mainland, D. (1971). Remarks on clinical "norms." *Clin. Chem.* 17, 267–274.

Manly, B. F. J. (1976). Exponential data transformations. *The Statistician* 25, 37–42.

Manzanares, C., Ibañez, A. Dorado, C. A., and Sanz, R. (1991). Theophylline concentrations predicted by the Chiou method. *Clin. Chem.* 37, 768–769.

Marks, V. (1985). A historical introduction. In *Therapeutic Drug Monitoring*, B. Widdop, ed. Churchill Livingstone, Edinburgh, pp. 3–15.

Martin, H. F., Gudzinowicz, B. J., and Fanger, H. (1975). *Normal Values in Clinical Chemistry*. Marcel Dekker, New York.

McCall, M. G. (1966). Normality. *J. Chron. Dis.* 19, 1127–1132.

McPherson, K., Healy, M. J. R., Flynn, F. V., et al. (1978). The effect of age, sex and other factors on blood chemistry in health. *Clin. Chim. Acta 84*, 373–397.

Meinhold, R. J., and Singpurwalla, N. D. (1983). Understanding the Kalman filter. *Amer. Statist.* 37, 123–127.

Meites, S., ed. (1989). *Pediatric Clinical Chemistry: Reference (Normal) Values*, 3rd ed. AACC Press, Washington, D.C.

Miller, W., Chinchilli, V. M., Gruemer, H.-D., and Nance, W. E. (1984). Sampling from a skewed population distribution as exemplified by estimation of the creatine kinase upper reference limit. *Clin. Chem. 30*, 18–23.

Milliken, G. A., and Johnson, D. E. (1984). *Analysis of Messy Data, Vol. 1: Designed Experiments.* Van Nostrand Reinhold, New York.

Mood, A. M. (1950). *Introduction to the Theory of Statistics.* McGraw-Hill, New York.

Moran P. A. P. (1968). *An Introduction to Probability Theory.* Oxford University Press, London.

Mosteller, F. (1946). On some useful "inefficient" statistics. *Ann. Math. Statist.* 17, 377–407.

Munan, L., Kelly, A., PetitClerc, C., and Billon, B. (1978). *Atlas of Blood Data.* Epidemiology Laboratory and Laboratory of Clinical Biochemistry, Faculty of Medicine, University of Sherbrooke, Quebec, Canada.

Murphy, E. A., and Abbey, H. (1967). The normal range: a common misuse. *J. Chron. Dis.* 20, 79–88.

Muth, J. F. (1960). Optimal properties of exponentially weighted forecasts. *J. Amer. Stat. Assoc.* 55, 297–306.

National Committee for Clinical Laboratory Standards (NCCLS) (1992). *How to Define, Determine, and Utilize Reference Intervals in the Clinical Laboratory, Proposed Guideline.* NCCLS Document C28-P. Villanova, PA.

Natrella, M. G. (1963). *Experimental Statistics.* National Bureau of Standards Handbook 91. U.S. Government Printing Office, Washington, D.C.

Neumann, G. J. (1968). The determination of normal ranges from routine laboratory data. *Clin. Chem.* 14, 979–988.

Nordic Clinical Chemistry Project (1980). *Assessing Quality Requirements in Clinical Chemistry,* M. Hørder, ed. Finnish Government Printing Center. Also published in *Scand. J. Clin. Lab. Invest.* 40 (Suppl. 155), 1980.

Nordic Clinical Chemistry Project (NORDKEM) (1984). *Optimized Use of Clinical Laboratory Data,* T. Groth, C.-H. De Verdier, and E. S. Benson, eds. Finnish Government Printing Center. Also published in *Scand. J. Clin. Lab. Invest.* 44 (Suppl. 171), 1984.

Nordic Clinical Chemistry Project (NORDKEM) (1992). *Some Concepts* and *Principles of Clinical Test Evaluation: Classification, Analytical Performance, Monitoring and Clinical Interpretation.* E. Magid, ed. Finnish Government Printing Center. Helsinki, Finland.

Nosanchuk, J. S., and Gottmann, A. W. (1974). CUMS and delta checks. *Am. J. Clin. Pathol. 62,* 707–712.

Oesterling, J. E., Jacobsen, S. J., Chute, C. G., et al. (1993). Serum prostate-specific antigen in a community-based population of healthy men. *J. Amer. Med. Assoc. 270,* 860–864.

O'Leary, P., Boyne, P., and Flett, P. (1991). Longitudinal assessment of changes in reproductive hormones during normal pregnancy. *Clin. Chem. 37,* 667–672.

Oosterhuis, W. P., Modderman, T. A., and Pronk, C. (1990). Reference values: Bhattacharya or the method proposed by the IFCC? *Ann. Clin. Biochem. 27,* 359–365.

Pan, H. Q., Goldstein, H., and Yang, Q. (1990). Non-parametric estimation of age-related centiles over wide age ranges. *Ann. of Human Biology 17,* 475–481.

Pantula, S. G. and Pollock, K. H. (1985). Nested analysis of variance with autocorrelated errors. *Biometrics 41,* 909–920.

Payne, R. B. and Levell, M. J. (1967). Redefinition of the normal range for serum calcium. *Clin. Chem. 14,* 172–178.

Petersen, P. H., and Hørder, M. (1988). Ways of assesssing quality goals for diagnostic tests in clinical situations. *Arch. Pathol. Lab. Med. 112,* 435–443.

Petersen, P. H., Gowans, E. M. S., Blaabjerg, O., and Hørder, M. (1989). Analytical goals for the estimation of non-Gaussian reference intervals. *Scand. J. Clin. Lab. Invest. 49,* 727–737.

Phillipou, G., and Phillips, P. J. (1993). Intraindividual variation of glycohemoglobin: implications for interpretation and analytical goals. *Clin. Chem. 39,* 2305–2308.

Pickup, J. F., Harris, E. K., Kearns, M. and Brown, S. S. (1977). Intraindividual variation of some serum constituents and its relevance to population-based reference ranges. *Clin. Chem. 23,* 842–850.

Potts, J. T. Jr., ed. (1991). Proceedings of the NIH Consensus Development Conference on Diagnosis and Management of Asymptomatic Primary Hyperparathyroidism. *J. Bone Miner. Res.* 6 (Suppl. 2).

Pryce, J. D. (1960). Level of haemoglobin in whole blood and red blood-cells, and proposed convention for defining normality. *Lancet* 2, 333–336.

Pryce, J. D. (1970). The normal range. *J. Amer. Med. Assoc.* 212, 883–884.

Queraltó, J. M., Boyd, J. C., and Harris, E. K. (1993). On the calculation of reference change values, with examples from a long-term study. *Clin. Chem.* 39, 1398–1403.

Raun, N. E., Møller, B. B., Back, U., and Gad, I. (1982). On individual reference intervals based on a longitudinal study of plasma proteins and lipids in healthy subjects, and their possible clinical application. *Clin. Chem.* 28, 294–300.

Recommendations for Improving Cholesterol Measurement: A Report from the Laboratory Standardization Panel of the National Cholesterol Education Program (1990). Public Health Service, U.S. Department of Health and Human Services, NIH Pub. No. 90-2964, Washington D.C.

Reed, A. H., (1970). Multitest screening and ninety-five percent limits. *Am. J. Clin. Path.* 54, 774–776.

Reed, A. H., and Wu, G. T. (1974). Evaluation of a transformation method for estimation of normal range. *Clin. Chem.* 20, 576-581.

Reed, A. H., Henry, R. J., and Mason, W. B. (1971). Influence of statistical method used on the resulting estimate of normal range. *Clin. Chem.* 17, 275–284.

Reed, A. H., Cannon, D. C., Winkelman, J. W., et al. (1972). Estimation of normal ranges from a controlled sample survey. I. Sex- and age-related influence on the SMA 12/60 screening group of tests. *Clin. Chem.* 18, 57–66.

Rehpenning, von W., Harm, K., Domesle, A., and Voigt, K. D. (1979). Falsch positive Werte bei der Vielfachanalyse: Die Abschätzung ihrer Häufigkeit mit der *Sylvester*chen Formel und ihre Reduktion durch eine multivariate Testgrösse. *J. Clin. Chem. Clin. Biochem. 17*, 565–572.

Report of the National Cholesterol Education Program Expert Panel on Detection, Evaluation, and Treatment of High Blood Cholesterol in Adults (1988). *Arch. Intern. Med. 148*, 36–69.

Roberts, L. B. (1967). The normal ranges with statistical analysis for seventeen blood constituents. *Clin. Chim. Acta 16*, 69–78.

Rode, R. A., and Chinchilli, V. M. (1988). The use of Box-Cox transformations in the development of multivariate tolerance regions with applications to clinical chemistry. *Amer. Statist. 42*, 23–30.

Rohatgi, V. K. (1984). *Statistical Inference.* Wiley, New York.

Rootwelt, K., and Solberg, H. E. (1981). Free thyroxine, thyroxine/TBG ratio and other *in vitro* tests of thyroid function evaluated by discriminant analysis. *Scand. J. Clin. Lab. Invest. 41*, 483–491.

Ross, J. W. (1982). Evaluation of precision. In *CRC Handbook of Clinical Chemistry,* Vol. 1, M. Werner, ed. CRC Press, Boca Raton, FL, pp. 391–422.

Ross, J. W. (1988). A theoretical basis for clinically relevant proficiency testing evaluation limits: sensitivity analysis of the effect of inherent test error upon acceptable method error. *Arch. Pathol. Lab. Med. 112*, 421–434.

Ross, J. W., and Tholen, D. W. (1987). Optimizing clinical laboratory analytic accuracy: a historical perpective, system analysis and model of clinical utility. In *Quality Assurance in Physician Office, Bedside and Home Testing,* P. J. Howanitz, ed. College of American Pathologists, Skokie, IL, pp. 85–125.

Ross, J. W., Fraser, M. D., and Moore, T. D. (1980). Analytic clinical laboratory precision: state of the art for thirty-one analytes. *Am. J. Clin. Pathol. 74*, 521–530.

Rossiter, J. E. (1991). Calculating centile curves using kernel density estimation methods with application to infant kidney lengths. *Statist. Med. 10*, 1693–1701.

Rotterdam, W. G. E., Kotan, M. B., and Knuiman, J. T. (1987). Importance of time interval between repeated measurements of total or high density lipoprotein cholesterol when estimating an individual's baseline concentrations. *Clin. Chem. 33*, 1913–1915.

Royston, J. P. (1982). An extension of Shapiro and Wilk's test for normality to large samples. *Appl. Statist. 31*, 115–124.

Royston, P. (1991). Constructing time-specific reference ranges. *Statist. Med. 10*, 675–690.

Royston, P. (1992). Estimation, reference ranges and goodness of fit for the three-parameter log-normal distribution. *Statist. Med. 11*, 897–912.

Sackett, D. L. (1973). Opinion: the usefulness of laboratory tests in health-screening programs. *Clin. Chem. 19*, 366–372.

Sanathanan, L. P., and Peck, C. C. (1991). The randomized concentration-controlled trial: an evaluation of its sample size efficiency. *Controlled Clin. Trials 12*, 780–794.

Sasaki, M. (1991) An innovative conveyor belt system for a clinical laboratory. *J. Int. Fed. Clin. Chem. 3*, 31–33.

Sasaki, M., and Ogura K. (1990) A fully robotic assay for human hormone analysis. *Clin. Chem. 36*, 1567–1571.

Savory, D. J. (1990). Reference ranges for serum creatinine in infants, children and adolescents. *Ann. Clin. Biochem. 27*, 99–101.

Schlain, B. R., Lavin, P. T., and Hayden, C.L. (1992). Using an autoregressive model to detect departures from steady states in unequally spaced tumor biomarker data. *Statist. Med. 11*, 515–532.

Schlain, B. R., Lavin, P. T., and Hayden, C. L. (1993). Using autoregressive and random walk models to detect trends and shifts in unequally spaced tumor biomarker data. *Statist. Med. 12*, 265–279.

Schneider, A. J. (1960). Some thoughts on normal, or standard, values in clinical medicine. *Pediatrics 26*, 973–984.

Schoen, I., and Brooks, S.H. (1970). Judgment based on 95% confidence limits: a statistical dilemma involving multitest screening and proficiency testing of multiple specimens. *Amer. J. Clin. Pathol. 53*, 190–193.

Schumacher, G. E., and Barr, J. T. (1989). Making serum drug levels more meaningful. *Therap. Drug Monit.* 11, 580–584.

Scott, J. E. S., Hunter, E. W., Lee, R. E. J., and Mathews, J. N. S., (1990). Ultrasound measurement of renal size in newborn infants. *Arch. Dis. Childhood* 65, 361–364.

Shahangian, S., Fritsche, Jr., H. A., Hughes, J. I., and Johnston, D.A. (1989). Methods for determining "reference changes" from serial measurements: plasma lipid-bound sialic acid. *Clin. Chem.* 35, 972–974.

Sheather, S. J., and Marron, J. S. (1990). Kernel quantile estimator. *J. Amer. Statist. Assoc.* 85, 410–416.

Sheehan, M., and Haythorn, P. (1979). Predictive values of various liver function tests with respect to the diagnosis of liver disease. *Clin. Chem.* 12, 262–263.

Sheiner, L. B., and Beal, S. L. (1982). Bayesian individualization of pharmacokinetics: simple implementation and comparison with non-Bayesian methods. *J. Pharmaceut. Sci.* 71, 1344–1348.

Sheiner, L. B., and Ludden, T. (1992). Population pharmacokinetics/ dynamics. *Annu. Rev. Pharmacol. Toxicol.* 32, 185–209.

Sheiner, L. B., Rosenberg, B., and Melmon, K. L. (1972). Modelling of individual pharmacokinetics for computer-aided drug dosage. *Comput. Biomed. Res.* 5, 441–459.

Sheiner, L. B., Rosenberg, B., and Marathe, V. V. (1977). Estimation of population characteristics of pharmacokinetic parameters from routine clinical data. *J. Pharmacokinet. Biopharmaceut.* 5, 445–479.

Sheiner, L. B., Wheeler, L. A., and Moore, J. K. (1979a). The performance of the delta check methods. *Clin. Chem.* 25, 2034–2037.

Sheiner, L. B., Beal, S., Rosenberg, B., and Marathe, V. V. (1979b). Forecasting individual pharmacokinetics. *Clin. Pharmacol. Ther.* 26, 294–305.

Sher, P. P. (1979). An evaluation of the detection capacity of a computer-assisted real-time delta check system. *Clin. Chem.* 25, 870–872.

Shultz, E. K., Willard, K. E., Rich, S. S. et al. (1985). Improved reference-interval estimation. *Clin. Chem.* 31, 1974–1978.

Shumway, R. H. (1988). *Applied Statistical Time Series Analysis*. Prentice-Hall, Englewood Cliffs, NJ.

Siest, G. (1981). Strategy for the establishment of healthy population reference values. In *Reference Values in Laboratory Medicine*, R. Gräsbeck and T. Alström, eds. Wiley, New York, pp. 45–53.

Siest, G., Henny, J., Schiele, F., and Young, D. S. (1985). *Interpretation of Clinical Laboratory Tests: Reference Values and Their Biological Variation*. Biomedical Publications, Foster City, CA.

Silverman, B. W. (1986). *Density Estimation for Statistics and Data Analysis*. Chapman & Hall, London.

Sinton, T. J., Cowley, D. M., and Bryant, S. J. (1986). Reference intervals for calcium, phosphate, and alkaline phosphatase as derived on the basis of multichannel-analyzer profiles. *Clin. Chem. 32*, 76–79.

Skendzel, L. P. (1978). How physicians use laboratory tests. *J. Amer. Med. Assoc. 239*, 1077–1080.

Skendzel, L. P., Barnett, R. P., and Platt, R. (1985). Medically useful criteria for analytic performance of laboratory tests. *Amer. J. Clin. Pathol. 83*, 200–205.

Smith, A. F. M., and West, M. (1983). Monitoring renal transplants: an application of the multiprocess Kalman filter. *Biometrics 39*, 867–878.

Smith, S. J., Cooper, G. R., Myers, G. L., and Sampson, E. J. (1993). Biological variability in concentrations of serum lipids: sources of variation among results from published studies and composite predicted values. *Clin. Chem. 39*, 1012–1022.

Solberg, H. E. (1983). REFVAL. A set of computer programs for the statistical treatment of reference values and the determination of reference limits. Technical Report, Department of Clinical Chemistry, Rikshospitalet, Oslo, Norway.

Solberg, H. E. (1985). Discriminant analysis. In *Handbook of Clinical Chemistry*, Vol. 3. Mario Werner, ed. CRC Press, Boca Raton, FL, pp. 215–245.

Solberg, H. E., and Gräsbeck, R. (1989). Reference values. *Adv. Clin. Chem. 27*, 1–79.

Solberg, H. E. Skrede, S., and Blomhoff, J. P. (1975). Diagnosis of liver diseases by laboratory results: identification of best combinations of laboratory tests. *Scand. J. Clin. Lab. Invest. 35*, 713–721.

Sölétormos, G., Schiøler, V., Nielsen, D., et al. (1993). Interpretation of results for tumor markers on the basis of analytical imprecision and biological variation. *Clin. Chem. 39*, 2077–2083.

Sox H. C. (1994). Practice guidelines: 1994. *Am. J. Med. 97*, 205–207.

Spyckerelle, Y., Steinmetz, J., and Deschamps, J. P. (1992). Comparaison à cinq ans d'intervalle des taux de cholestérol, glucose et acide urique chez l'enfant et l'adolescent. *Arch. Fr. Pediatr. 9*, 875–881.

Statland, B. E., (1987). *Clinical Decision Levels for Lab Tests*, 2nd ed. Medical Economics, Oradell, NJ.

Statland, B. E., and Winkel, P. (1977). Effects of non-analytical factors on the intra-individual variation of analytes in the blood of healthy subjects: consideration of preparation of the subject and time of venipuncture. *CRC Crit. Rev. Clin. Lab. Sci. 8*, 105–144.

Statland, B. E., and Winkel, P. (1981). Selected pre-analytical sources of variation. In *Reference Values in Laboratory Medicine*, R. Gräsbeck and T. Alström, eds. Wiley, New York, pp. 127–137.

Statland, B. E., Winkel, P., and Bokelund, H. (1973). Factors contributing to intra-individual variation of serum constituents: 2. Effects of exercise and diet on variation of serum constituents in healthy subjects. *Clin. Chem. 19*, 1380–1383.

Statland, B. E., Bokelund, H., and Winkel, P. (1974). Factors contributing to intra-individual variation of serum constituents: 4. Effects of posture and tourniquet application on variation of serum constituents in healthy subjects. *Clin. Chem. 20*, 1513–1519.

Statland, B. E., Winkel, P., and Killingsworth, L. M. (1976). Factors contributing to intra-individual variation of serum constituents: 6. Physiological day-to-day variation in concentrations of 10 specific proteins in sera of healthy subjects. *Clin. Chem. 22*, 1635–1638.

Stewart, K. B. (1970). A new weighted average. *Technometrics 12*, 247–258.

Sunderman, Jr., F. W. (1970). Expected distributions of normal and abnormal results in multitest surveys of healthy subjects. *Amer. J. Clin. Pathol.* 53, 288–291.

Sunderman, Jr., F. W. (1975). Current concepts of "normal values," "reference values," and "discrimination values" in clinical chemistry. *Clin. Chem.* 21, 1873–1877.

Tamura, M., Inasaki, M., Ohno, H., and Kitaike, T. (1987). Principles learned from 15 years' experience in long-term monitoring of individual subjects in a health maintenance program. In *Maintaining a Healthy State Within the Individual*, E.K. Harris and T. Yasaka, eds. Elsevier/North-Holland, Amsterdam, pp. 9–25.

Taylor, D. R., Kinney, C. D., and McDevitt, D. G. (1984). Patient compliance with oral theophylline therapy. *Br. J. Clin. Pharmacol.* 17, 15–20.

Taylor, L. R. (1961). Aggregation, variance and the mean. *Nature (Lond.)* 189, 732–735.

Thienpont, L. M. R., Steyaert, H. L. C., and DeLeenheer, A. P. (1987). A modified statistical approach for the detection of outlying values in external quality control: comparison with other techniques. *Clin. Chim. Acta* 168, 337–346.

Thue, G., Sandberg, S., and Fugelli P. (1991). Clinical assessment of haemoglobin values by general practitioners related to analytical and biological variation. *Scand. J. Clin. Lab. Invest.* 51, 453–459.

Tietz, N. W. (1979). A model for a comprehensive measurement system in clinical chemistry. *Clin. Chem.* 25, 833–839.

Tonks, D. B. (1963). A study of the accuracy and precision of clinical chemistry in 170 Canadian laboratories. *Clin. Chem.* 9, 217–233.

Tukey, J. W. (1977). *Exploratory Data Analysis.* Addison-Wesley, Reading, MA.

Ueland, P. M., Refsum, H., Stabler, S. P., et al. (1993). Total homocysteine in plasma or serum: methods and clinical applications. *Clin. Chem.* 39, 1764–1779.

Van Der Meulen, E. A., Boogaard, P. J., and Van Sittert, N. J. (1994). Use of small-sample-based reference limits on a group basis. *Clin. Chem.* 40, 1698–1702.

van Dobben de Bruyn, C. S. (1968). *Cumulative Sum Tests: Theory and Practice*. Griffin, London.

Van Peenen, H. J., and Lindberg, D. A. B. (1965). Limitations of laboratory quality control with reference to the "number plus" method. *Amer. J. Clin. Pathol. 44*, 322–330.

Van Steirteghem, A. C., Robertson, E. A., and Young, D. S. (1978). Variance components of serum constituents in healthy individuals. *Clin. Chem. 24*, 212–222.

van't Hof, M. A., Wit, J. M., and Roede, M. J. (1985). A method to construct age references for skewed skinfold data, using Box-Cox transformations to normality. *Hum. Biol. 57*, 131–139.

Voisin, E. M., Ruthsatz, M., Collins, J. M., and Hoyle, P. C. (1990). Extrapolation of animal toxicity to humans: interspecies comparisons in drug development. *Regul. Toxicol. Pharmacol. 12*, 107–116.

von Neumann, J. (1941). Distribution of the ratio of the mean square successive difference to the variance. *Ann. Math. Statist. 12*, 307–395.

Vožeh S., and Steimer, J.-L. (1985). Feedback control methods for drug dosage optimization: concepts, classification and clinical application. *Clin. Pharmacokinet. 10*, 457–476.

Ware, J. H. (1985). Linear models for the analysis of longitudinal studies. *Amer. Statist. 39*, 95–101.

Weldon, K. L., and MacKay, J. S. (1972a). On improving the diagnostic value of quantitative medical laboratory tests in conventional practice. *J. Chron. Dis. 25*, 683–696.

Weldon, K. L., and MacKay, J. S. (1972b). On improving the diagnostic value of quantitative medical laboratory tests in health screening. *J. Chron. Dis. 25*, 697–709.

Welling, P. G. (1986). *Pharmacokinetics: Processes and Mathematics*. ACS Monograph 185. American Chemical Society, Washington, D.C.

Werner, M., Tolls, R. E., Hultin, J. V., and Mellecker, J. (1970). Influence of sex and age on the normal range of eleven serum constituents. *Z. Klin. Chem. Klin. Biochem. 8*, 105–115.

Westgard, J. O., and Barry P. L. (1986). *Cost-effective Quality Control:*

Managing the Quality and Productivity of Analytical Processes. American Association for Clinical Chemistry, Washington, D.C.

Westgard, J. O., and Burnett, R. W. (1990). Precision requirements for cost-effective operation of analytical processes. *Clin. Chem.* 36, 1629–1632.

Westgard, J. O., and Groth, T. (1979). Power functions for statistical control rules. *Clin. Chem.* 25, 863–869.

Westgard, J. O., Carey, R. N., and Wold, S. (1974). Criteria for judging precision and accuracy in method development and evaluation. *Clin. Chem.* 20, 825–833.

Westgard, J. O., Groth, T., Aronsson, T., and deVerdier, C.-H. (1977). Combined Shewhart-Cusum control chart for improved quality control in clinical chemistry. *Clin. Chem.* 23, 1881–1887.

Westgard, J. O., Petersen, P. H., and Wiebe, D. A. (1991). Laboratory process specifications for assuring quality in the U.S. National Cholesterol Education Program. *Clin. Chem.* 37, 656–661.

Wheeler, L. A., and Sheiner, L. B. (1977). Delta check tables for the Technicon SMA 6 continuous-flow analyzer. *Clin. Chem.* 23, 216–219.

Wheeler, L. A., and Sheiner, L. B. (1981). A clinical evaluation of various delta check methods. *Clin. Chem.* 27, 5–9.

Whitehurst P., DiSilvio, T. V., and Boyadjian, G. (1975). Evaluation of discrepancies in patients' results: an aspect of computer-assisted quality control. *Clin. Chem.* 21, 87–92.

Whiting, B, Kelman, A. W., and Grevel J. (1986). Population pharmacokinetics theory and clinical application. *Clin. Pharmacokinet.* 11, 387–401.

Wilding, P., Rollason, J. G., and Robinson, D. (1972). Patterns of change for various biochemical constituents detected in well population screening. *Clin. Chim. Acta* 41, 375–387.

Wilks, S. S. (1963). Multivariate statistical outliers. *Sankhyā A25,* 407–426.

Williams, G. Z. (1962). Clinical pathology tomorrow. *Amer. J. Clin. Pathol.* 37, 121–124.

Williams, G. Z. (1967). Individuality of clinical biochemical patterns in preventive health maintenance. *J. Occup. Med. 9,* 567–570.

Williams, G. Z. (1993). Serum lipid values and age in healthy women: a preliminary report on cholesterol. *Meth. Inform. Med. 32,* 219–221.

Williams, G. Z., Harris, E. K., and Widdowson, G. M. (1977). Comparison of estimates of long-term analytical variation derived from subject samples and control serum. *Clin. Chem. 23,* 100–104.

Williams, G. Z., Widdowson, G. M., and Penton, J. (1978). Individual character of variation in time-series studies of healthy people. II. Differences in values for clinical chemical analytes in serum among demographic groups, by age and sex. *Clin. Chem. 24,* 313–320.

Williams, G. Z., Young, D. S., Stein, M. R., and Cotlove, E. (1970). Biological and analytic components of variation in long-term studies of serum constituents in normal subjects. I. Objectives, subject-selection, laboratory procedures, and estimation of analytic deviation. *Clin. Chem. 16,* 1016–1021.

Williams, R. J. (1956). *Biochemical Individuality.* University of Texas Press, Austin.

Williams, R. J., Brown, W. D., and Shideler, R. W. (1955). Metabolic peculiarities in normal young men as revealed by repeated blood analyses. *Proc. NAS 41,* 615–620.

Winkel, P., Gaede P., and Lyngbye J. (1976). Method for monitoring plasma progesterone concentrations in pregnancy. *Clin. Chem. 22,* 422–428.

Winkel, P., Lyngbye, J., and Jörgensen, K. (1972). The normal region: a multivariate problem. *Scand. J. Clin. Lab. Invest. 30,* 339–344.

Winkel, P., Statland, B. E., and Bokelund, H. (1975). The effects of time of venipuncture on variation of serum constituents: consideration of within-day and day-to-day changes in a group of healthy young men. *Amer. J. Clin. Pathol. 64,* 433–437.

Winkel, P., Bentzon, M. W., Statland, B. E., et al. (1982). Predicting recurrence in patients with breast cancer from cumulative laboratory results: a new technique for the application of time series analysis. *Clin. Chem. 28,* 2057–2067.

Winkelman, J. W., Cannon, D. C., Pileggi, V. J., and Reed, A. H. (1973). Estimation of norms from a controlled sample survey. II. Influence of body habitus, oral contraceptives, and other factors on values for the normal range derived from the SMA 12/60 screening group of tests. *Clin. Chem. 19*, 488–491.

Wong, E. T., Cobb, C., Umehara, M.K., et al. (1983). Heterogeneity of serum creatine kinase activity among racial and gender groups of the population. *Amer. J. Clin. Pathol. 79*, 582–586.

Woolf, S. H. (1993). Practice guidelines: a new reality in medicine. III. Impact on patient care. *Arch. Intern. Med. 153*, 2646–2655.

Wootton, I. D. P. (1962). Individual variation. *Proc. Nutr. Soc. 21*, 129–135.

Wootton, I. D. P., and King, E. J. (1953). Normal values for blood constituents. *Lancet 264*, 470–471.

Wootton, I. D. P., King, E. J., and Smith, J. M. (1951). The quantitative approach to hospital biochemistry. *Br. Med. Bull. 7*, 307–311.

World Association of Societies of Pathology (1979). Analytical goals in clinical chemistry: their relationship to medical care. Proceedings of a subcommittee. *Amer. J. Clin. Pathol. 7*, 624–630.

Yasaka, T., Nakano, K., and Mizunuma, T. (1978). Clinical data evaluation and the PL health control information system. *Comput. Programs Biomed. 8*, 51–70.

Yaschin, E. (1985). On the analysis and design of CUSUM-Shewhart control schemes. *IBM J. Res. Devel. 29*, 377–391.

Young, D. S. (1990). *Effects of Drugs on Clinical Laboratory Tests*, 3rd ed. AACC Press, Washington, D.C.

Young, D. S. (1993). *Effect of Preanalytical Variables on Clinical Laboratory Tests*. American Association for Clinical Chemistry, Washington, D.C.

Young D. S., Harris, E. K., and Cotlove, E. (1971). Biological and analytic components of variation in long-term studies of serum constituents in normal subjects. IV. Results of a study designed to eliminate long-term analytic deviations. *Clin. Chem. 17*, 403–410.

INDEX